ATLAS
OF
REARFOOT SURGERY

ATLAS OF REARFOOT SURGERY

Louis J. Arancia, D.P.M., F.A.C.F.S.

Fellow, American College of Foot Surgeons
Diplomate, American Board Podiatric Surgery
Director of Podiatric Surgery, Baptist Hospital of New York, Brooklyn, New York

Frank T. Rinaldi, D.P.M., F.A.C.F.O.

Fellow, American College of Foot Orthopedists
Board Eligible, American Board Podiatric Surgery
Director of Education, First and Second Year Podiatric Surgical Residency Programs, Baptist Hospital of New York, Brooklyn, New York

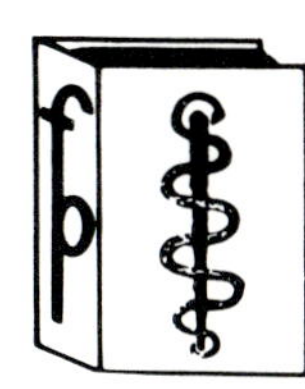

FUTURA PUBLISHING COMPANY, INC.
MOUNT KISCO, NEW YORK
1978

Published by
Futura Publishing Company, Inc.
P.O. Box 298, 295 Main Street
Mount Kisco, New York 10549

L.C. #: 78-67922
ISBN #: 0-87993-095-0

Printed in U.S.A.

Dedication

This book is dedicated to our families —
Elaine, Carol, Frances, and John Arancia,
Marie, Thomas, and Betty Rinaldi.
For their love and devotion
we thank them.

Preface

This book is the first extensive effort to correlate, in atlas form, surgery of the rearfoot. Excellent medical literature dealing with parts or different aspects of our subject matter has been published, but none has attempted to embrace or encompass the entire field. We therefore undertook this task to guide the student, the general practitioner, and the surgeon of the foot through the maze of procedures that can be performed on the rearfoot.

The eclectic nature of the material we have gathered is evident by the long bibliographies. Our aim was to research and digest the voluminous literature and provide the reader with the most significant procedures performed on the hindfoot; although some surely must have escaped our notice. However, in our zeal to be complete, we have included surgeries whose values are more facultative and historical than frequently performed.

One should not consider this work to be encyclopedic in scope; rather it is an atlas for those desirous of up-to-date coverage of the subject. The book is divided into chapters that contain diagrammatic illustrations and analytical descriptions of surgical procedures for specific conditions. The reader will find the introductory text concise and informative.

We wish to extend our sincere gratitude to the many publishers who gave permission and materials for illustrations. We would also like to thank Dr. Nicholas Aloi for planting the seed for this endeavor. Our special thanks go out to our secretaries, Mrs. Audrey Nardone and Miss Carol Arancia for typing and retyping this manuscript.

Contents

CHAPTER 1

Haglund's Disease

Haglund's disease, also known as "retrocalcaneal bursitis" or "pump bump", is characterized by an exostosis on the posterosuperior aspect of the heel, associated with tenderness and localized inflammation. This acquired deformity is most common among adolescent females, but it can affect people of either sex at any age.

The retrocalcaneal prominence in Haglund's disease is commonly thought to be secondary to mechanical friction, generally between a short shoe counter and the prominent superior edge of the calcaneus in the region of the attachment of the tendo Achillis. The heel counter of the standard shoe, designed to fit a convex surface, does not always fit the contour of the posterosuperior edge of the calcaneus. Over time, incorrect fit at the heel can lead to the development of Haglund's disease—often of both feet.

Fowler and Philip have studied retrocalcaneal bursitis in terms of possible causes. In their clinical investigations they were able to demonstrate that in the normal foot the angle of the calcaneus from its posterior aspect to its plantar surface is in the range of 44 degrees to 62 degrees. Among patients with Haglund's disease, however, this angle was greater than 75 degrees in every case.[1]

Knowledge of the Fowler-Philip angle is helpful in the diagnosis of a Haglund's deformity, but other factors have also been implicated. In contemplating surgical correction of the characteristic deformity of Haglund's disease, the foot surgeon should consider whether there is any abnormal motion compensating for a plantar-flexed digital ray or for rearfoot varus or forefoot valgus. Such compensation will invert the heel and can contribute to the exaggerated Fowler-Philip angle by creating a shearing pronatory force at the posterosuperior edge of the calcaneus. It is important to recognize that the degree of calcaneal angulation is in direct relation to the extent of the Haglund's disease, and therefore, all compensating forces, as well as mechanical friction, must be evaluated if a proper diagnosis is to be made.

When all possible causes have been evaluated and a course of conservative therapy has failed, corrective surgery is indicated.

Of the techniques illustrated here, the procedures developed by Keck and Kelly and by DuVries were designed to reduce the angle between the posterior calcaneus and its plantar surface from greater than 75 degrees to 62 degrees (upper range of normal). It should be noted that the Fowler-Philip technique was developed for removal of a retrocalcaneal bursa and is modified here to show the procedure for correction of the calcaneal hyperconvexity.

Posterosuperior Tuberosity of the Calcaneus

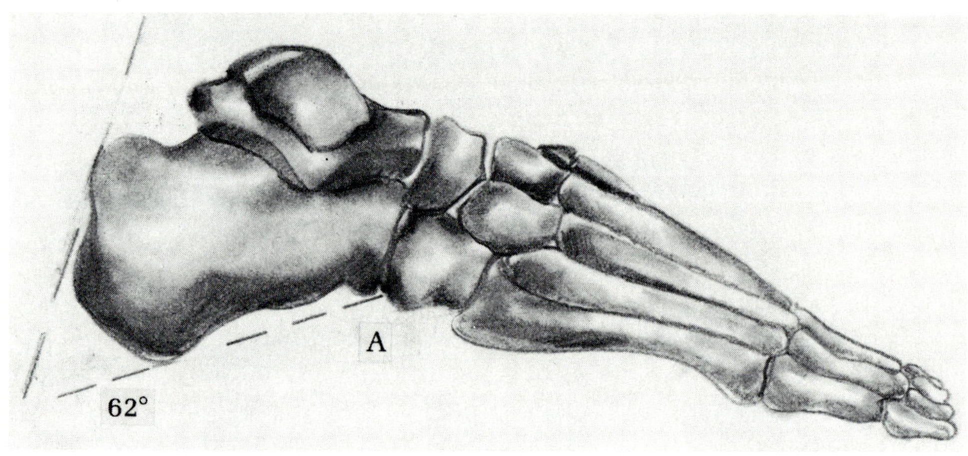

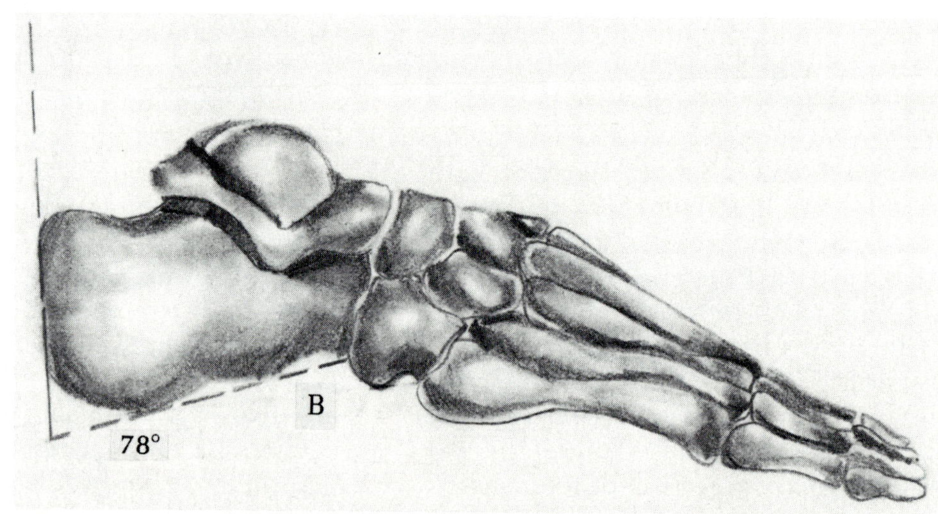

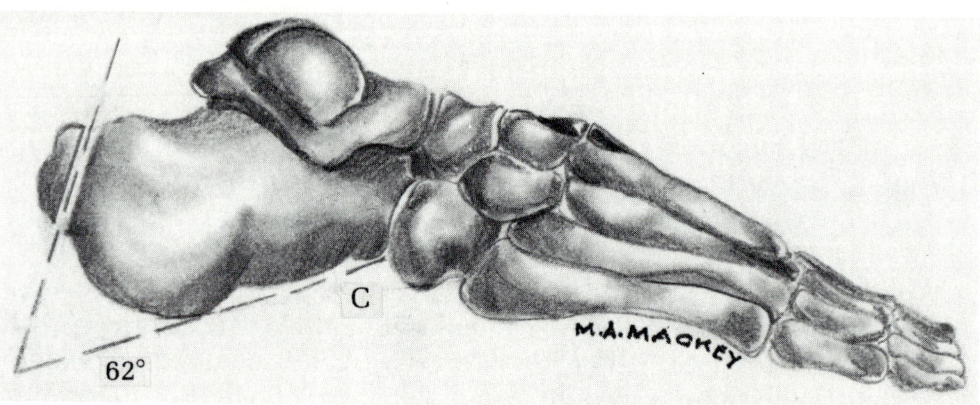

Figure 1. Posterosuperior tuberosity of the calcaneus. (A) Normal. (B) Prominent posterosuperior tuberosity. (C) Prominent tuberosity excised.

Fowler and Philip Excision of a Retrocalcaneal Bursa[2]

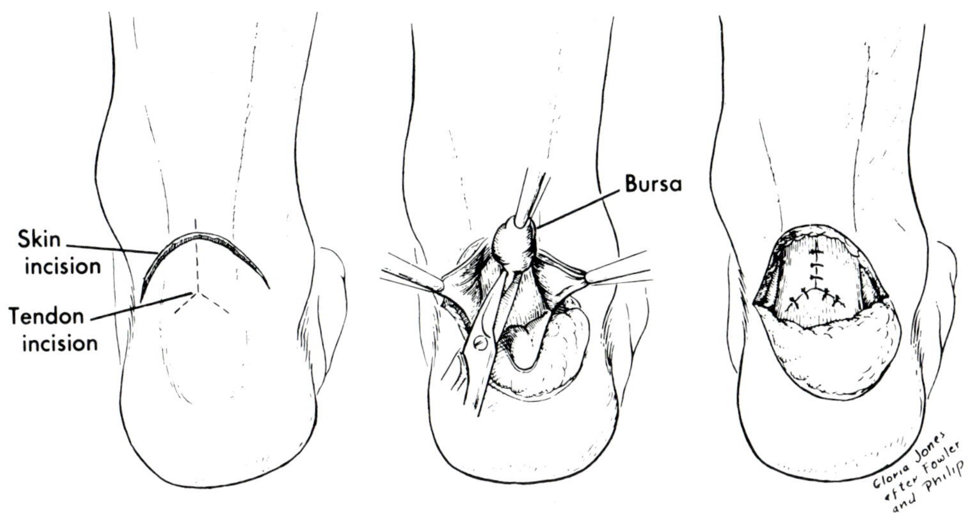

Figure 2. (Reproduced with permission from DuVries, H.L.: *Surgery of the Foot,* 2 ed., C.V. Mosby, St. Louis, 1965, p. 226.)

1. Semi-elliptical skin incision.
2. Inverted Y incision in the tendo Achillis.
3. Retrocalcaneal bursa dissected free and excised.
4. *Modification.* Exostosis removed.
5. Tendo Achillis sutured.
6. Skin closure effected.

Osteotomy to Decrease Prominence of Calcaneus[3] (Keck and Kelly)

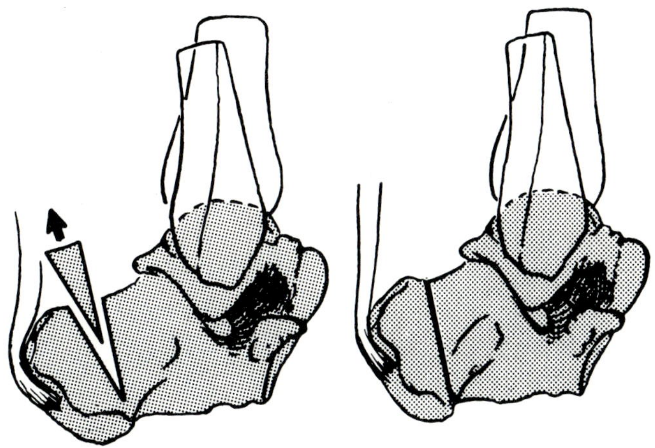

Figure 3. (Reproduced with permission from Inman, V.T. (Ed.): *DuVries' Surgery of the Foot,* 3 ed., C.V. Mosby, St. Louis, 1973, p. 495.)

1. Straight lateral skin incision at the terminal end of the tendo Achillis.
2. Excision of wedge-shaped piece of bone.
3. Rotation of the posterior portion of the calcaneus for mechanical reduction of the prominence at the posterosuperior margin of the bone near the attachment of the tendo Achillis.
4. Insertion of Steinmann pin, skin closure effected, and plaster of Paris cast applied with the foot in dorsiflexion to maintain apposition for six weeks.

DuVries Excision of Prominence of Calcaneus Through Lateral Incision[3]

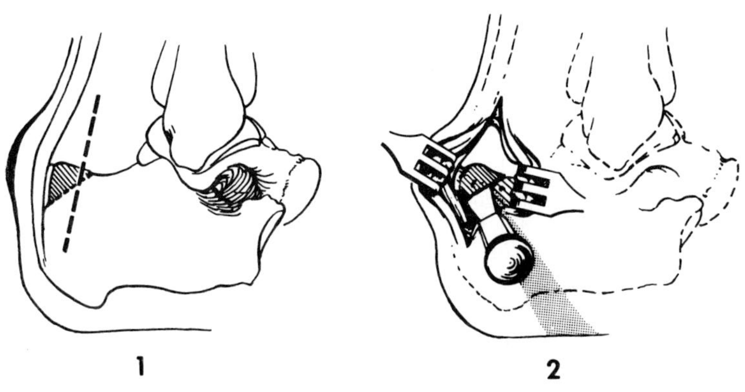

Figure 4. (Reproduced with permission from Inman, V.T. (Ed.): *DuVries' Surgery of the Foot,* 3 ed., C.V. Mosby, St. Louis, 1973, p. 494.)

1. A longitudinal incision approximately 7–8 cm long is made over the fibular aspect of the terminal end of the tendo Achillis.
2. Skin edges are undermined and retracted.
3. Longitudinal incision is made in the fibular side of the sheath of the tendo Achillis.
4. Weidtlander retractor inserted and posterosuperior edge of calcaneus exposed. Foot is held in plantar flexion so that the tendo Achillis is removed from the bone.
5. Osseous hypertrophy is excised by hammer and chisel and the cut edge rounded. Care should be taken to remove the excised hypertrophic bone laterally to medially to avoid injury to the posterior tibial bundle.
6. Area flushed with normal saline solution.
7. Tendon sheath sutured.
8. Subcutaneous and skin closures effected.

References

1. Fowler, A., and Philip, J.F.: Abnormality of calcaneus as cause of painful heel. *Br. J. Surg.*, **32**:494–498, 1945.
2. DuVries, H.L.: *Surgery of the Foot,* 2 ed., C.V. Mosby, St. Louis, 1965, pp. 224–228.
3. Inman, V.T. (Ed.): *DuVries' Surgery of the Foot,* 3 ed., C.V. Mosby, St. Louis, 1973, pp. 491–495.

Selected Bibliography

Keck, S.W., and Kelly, P.J.: Bursitis of the posterior part of the heel: evaluation of surgical treatment of eighteen patients. *J. Bone Jt. Surg.*, **47-A**:267–273, 1965.

Kelikan, H.: *Hallux Valgus, Allied Deformities of the Forefoot and Metatarsalgia,* W. B. Saunders, Philadelphia, 1965.

Ruch, J.A.: Haglund's Disease. J. Am. Pod. Assoc. **64**:1000–1003, 1974.

Sgarlato, T.E.: *A Compendium of Podiatric Biomechanics*, California College of Podiatric Medicine, San Francisco, 1971.

CHAPTER 2

Inferior Calcaneal Spur

Calcaneal spurs most commonly develop on the inferior medial surface of the calcaneus in the region of the origin of the plantar fascia. A typical symptom is pain in the heel at the beginning of walking, with gradual lessening of pain as walking continues; rest provides relief.

Spurs vary greatly in size and in shape, but most have a triangular form. A mediolateral, two-dimensional roentgenogram will reveal a tack-like protrusion, but spurs actually extend across the entire calcaneal tuberosity.

From early in the twentieth century there has been controversy about the origins of calcaneal spurs. In 1906 Baer postulated that they develop secondary to gonorrhea, and the term "gonorrheal heel" gained acceptance.[1] This theory was challenged in 1939 by Hauser, who suggested a mechanical cause from the "constant pull of a fascial or muscular attachment" to the calcaneus.[2] DuVries[3] and other investigators apparently agreed with the Hauser theory, but none stated a probable cause of the "constant pull". In 1949 Lewin offered various causes of calcaneal spurs, including focal injections, metabolic disturbances, trauma, and flat feet.[4] By 1954, however, Hicks[5] gave Hauser's theory credibility when he equated the action of the plantar fascia where it proceeds under the metatarsal heads to the function of a windlass. He stated that any abnormal motion causing pronation of the subtalar joint to the extent that the midtarsal joint is unlocked forces the foot to elongate. This lengthening subjects the calcaneal attachment of the plantar fascia to extreme stress.

Spur development is thought to begin with subperiosteal hemorrhage secondary to plantar fascial stress. Hemorrhage is followed by ingrowth of connective tissue fibers—a physiological response to the localized stress. The fibers initially are cartilaginous but gradually thicken and eventually become calcified to form the bony spur. Although there is not complete agreement that this is the exact mechanism of production of calcaneal spurs, most investigators agree that they are the result of mechanical stress.

The procedures for removal of spurs described here were developed by Griffith,[6] by Steindler,[7] and by DuVries.[8] In 1911 Griffith proposed his method in which a U-shaped incision is made around the entire heel so that the plantar surface can be reflected distally for access to the spur. Steindler's rotation osteotomy and the DuVries procedure are indicated in cases of recurrent calcaneal spurs; both techniques are designed to change the contact point of the os calcis. The change in the contact point serves to redistribute body weight toward the posterior surface of the heel in order to reduce focus on the stress point. DuVries' procedure is simpler and less traumatic than either Griffith's or Steindler's.

Spur Extends Over the Entire Width of the Tuberosity[3]

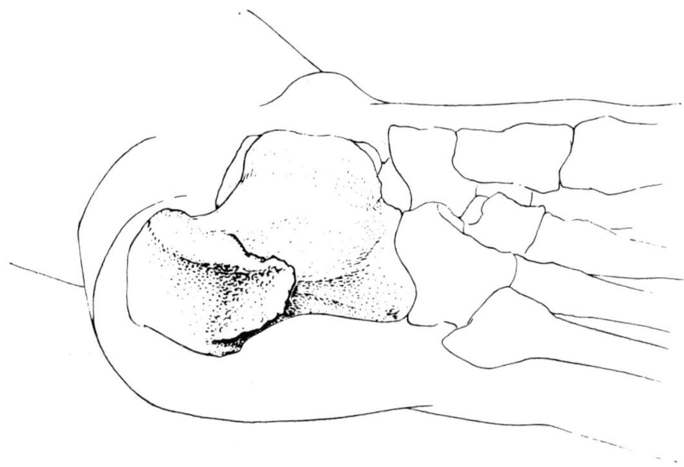

Figure 1. (Reproduced with permission from DuVries, H.L.: Heel spur (calcaneal spur), *Arch. Surg.*, **74**:536, 1957.)

Griffith's Procedure[3]

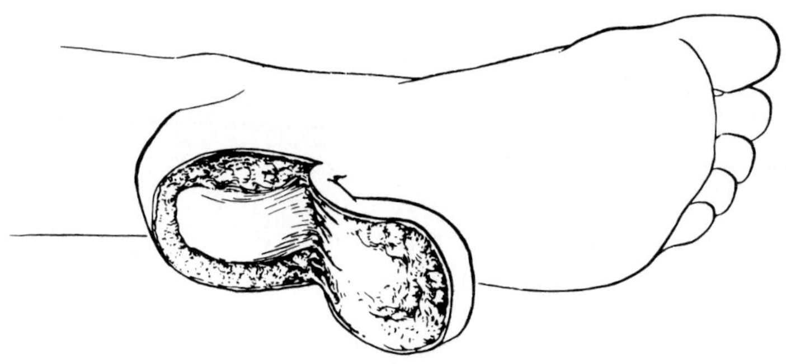

Figure 2. Entire plantar surface of the heel is denuded as a flap; the spur is removed; and then the flap is sutured into place. (Reproduced with permission from DuVries, H.L.: Heel spur (calcaneal spur), *Arch. Surg.*, **74**:536, 1957.)

1. U-shaped skin incision completely around the heel.
2. Skin flap denuded and reflected to expose the plantar surface of calcaneus.
3. Fascia severed at its origin and spur removed.
4. Flap sutured.

Rotation Osteotomy of Os Calcis for Calcaneal Spurs (Steindler's Method)[8]

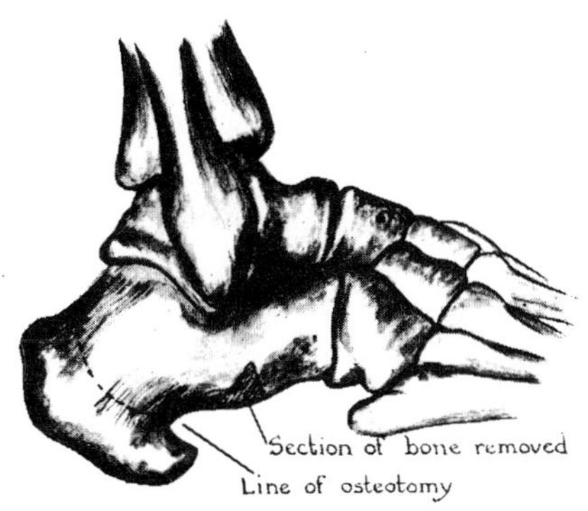

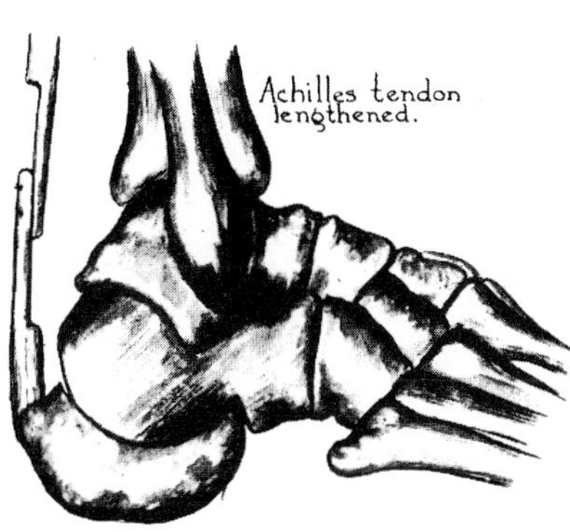

Figure 3. (Reproduced with permission from Steindler, A.: *Orthopedic Operations: Indications, Technique, and End Results,* Charles C Thomas, Springfield, Ill., 1940, p. 217.)

1. Tendo Achillis lengthened from posterior skin incision.
2. Short longitudinal incision made at the outer edge of the os calcis.
3. Os calcis freed from surrounding tissue through small internal incision made parallel with upper border of posterior process. Os calcis stripped from the periosteum on the inner side.
4. Arcular osteotomy made in the os calcis from the front of the tendo Achillis to the lower surface of the os calcis, approximately 1 inch further distally.
5. Groove chiseled in the body of the os calcis to receive the anterior edge of the posterior fragment.
6. Posterior fragment rotated approximately 90 degrees until its forward point fits into the chiseled groove.
7. The foot is placed into a slight equinus position, at which angle the os calcis is fixed with either a bone peg or a steel pin.
8. Plaster of Paris cast applied to maintain apposition for six to eight weeks. Walking on the toes is permitted after six weeks.

Excision of Calcaneal Spur (DuVries Procedure)

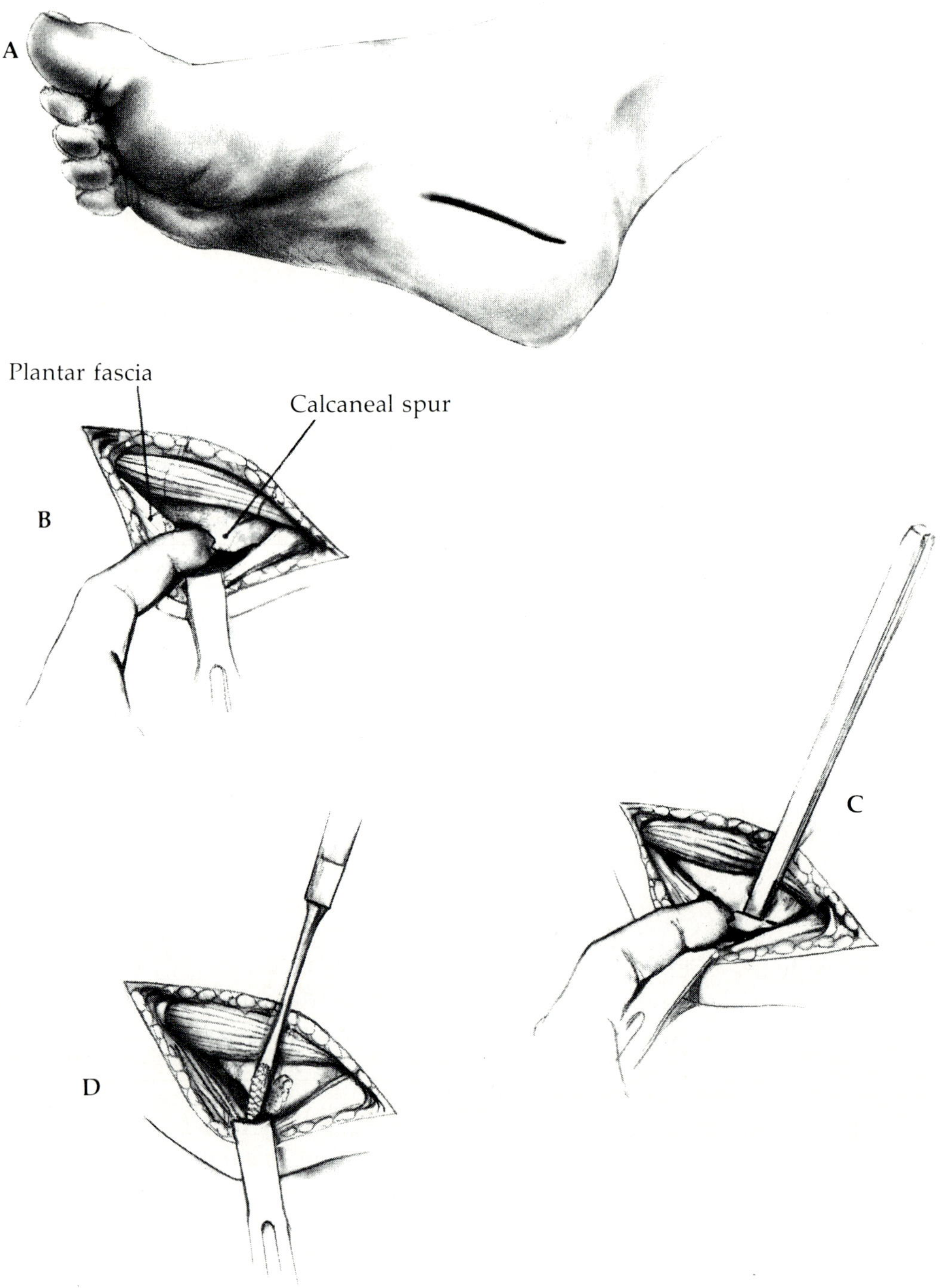

Figure 4. (Reproduced with permission from Goldstein, L.A., and Dickerson, R.C.: *Atlas of Orthopaedic Surgery*, Vol. 2, C.V. Mosby, St. Louis, 1974, p. 909.)

1. Linear skin incision approximately 6 cm in length made on the medial side of the heel above the plantar border.
2. DuVries stated that it is then possible to free the space immediately above the plantar fascia and the apex of the spur. In our experience this is not so; rather, the incision must be deepened and the abductor hallucis muscle incised.
3. Weidtlander retractor placed into the incision and opened to expose a hollow space through which the spur may be visualized.
4. Spur observed *above* the plantar fascia; not attached to it, as is stated in many textbooks.
5. With a sharp periosteal elevator, the spur is freed from filaments of the plantar fascia that adhere to it.
6. DuVries stated that it is possible to remove the spur with hand and osteotome by exerting palmar pressure. We have not found this to be practicable and therefore recommend use of the osteotome and hammer in spur removal.
7. DuVries recommended smoothing the surface of the calcaneus with a Joseph nasal rasp after excision of the spur. We do not agree with this approach, because rasping the cut surface can produce postoperative periosteal pain that will prolong incapacitation.
8. Flush area with normal saline solution.
9. Abductor hallucis muscle sutured with No. 3-0 Dexon®.
10. Fascia closed with No. 3-0 Dexon®.
11. Skin closure effected by subcuticular suturing with No. 3-0 wire.
12. Wire sutures are removed two to three weeks following operation.
13. Walking is permitted after four days, but physiotherapy is necessary for approximately six weeks. Use of a plastic heel cup is recommended until the patient is pain free.

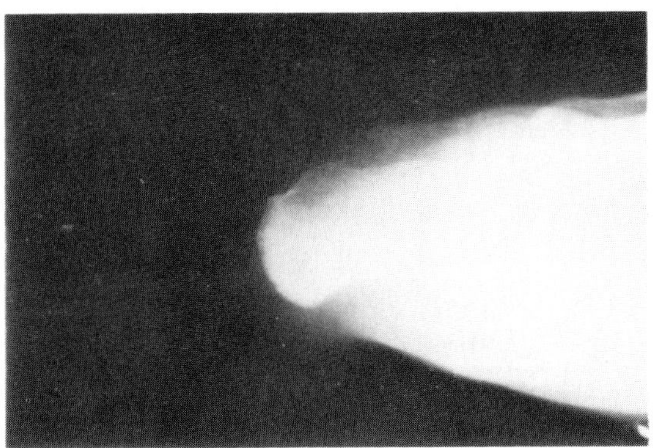
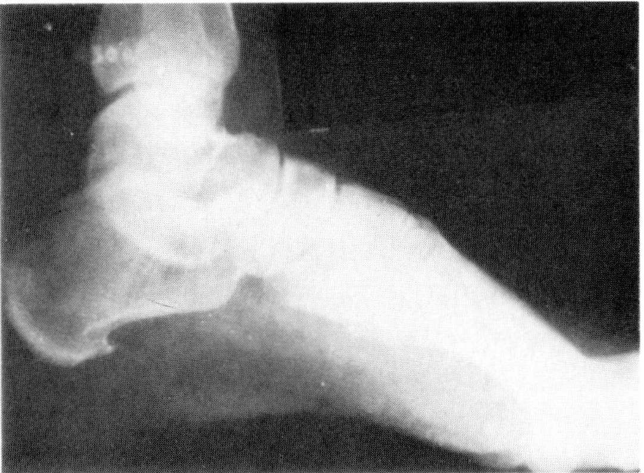

Figure 5. Calcaneal spur, preoperative.

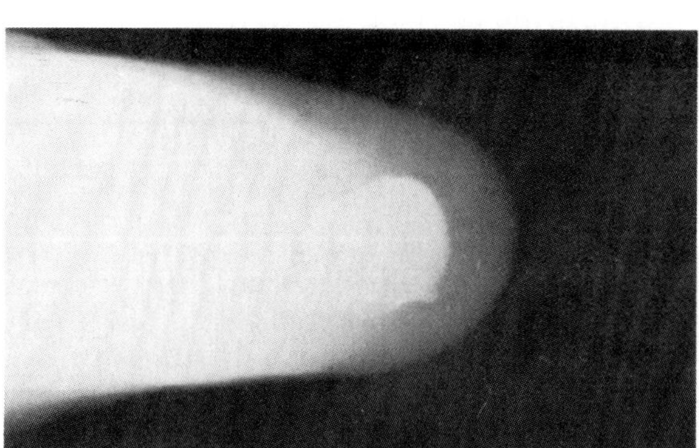

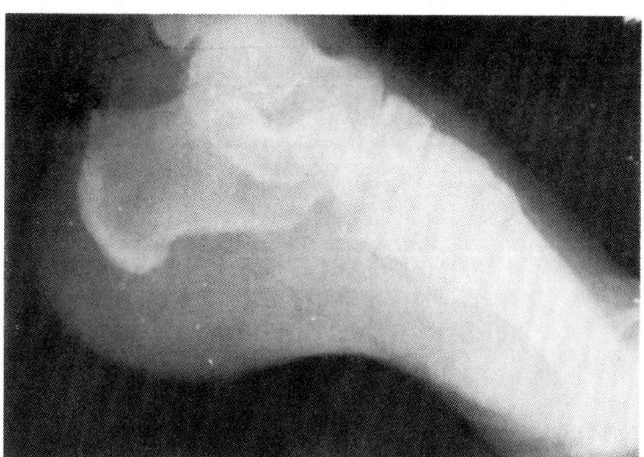

Figure 6. Calcaneal spur, 18 days postoperative.

References

1. Baer, W.S.: Painful Heels. *Bull. Johns Hopkins Hosp.*, **16**:264, 1906.
2. Hauser, E.: *Diseases of the Foot*, W.B. Saunders Co., Philadelphia, 1939.
3. DuVries, H.L.: Heel spur (calcaneal spur). *A.M.A. Arch. Surg.*, **74**:536, 1957.
4. Lewin, P.: *The Foot and Ankle*, 4 ed., Lea and Febiger, Philadelphia, 1959.
5. Hicks, J.H.: Mechanics of the foot: the plantar aponeurosis and the arch. *J. Anat.*, **88**:25, 1954.
6. Griffith, J.D.: Osteophytes of the os calcis. *Am. J. Orthop.*, **8**:501–506, Fed. 1010. p. 216–217.
7. Steindler, A., and Smith, A.R.: Spurs of the os calcis. *Surg. Gynecol. Obstet.*, **66**:663–665, 1938.
8. Steindler, A.: *Orthopaedic Operations*, Charles C Thomas, Springfield, Ill., 1940.

Selected Bibliography

Contompasis, J.P.: Surgical treatment of calcaneal spurs, *J. Am. Pod. Assoc.*, **64**:987–999, 1974.

Duggar, G.E.: Plantar fascitis and heel spurs. In E.D. McGlamry (Ed.): *Reconstructive Surgery of the Foot and Leg*, Intercontinental Medical Book Corporation, New York, 1974.

DuVries, H.L.: *Surgery of the Foot*, 2 ed., C.V. Mosby, St. Louis, 1965, pp. 158–168.

Goldstein, L.A., and Dickerson, R.C.: *Atlas of Orthopaedic Surgery*, Vol. 2, C.V. Mosby, St. Louis, 1974, pp. 908–909.

Lewin, P.: *The Foot and Ankle*, 4 ed., Lea & Febiger, Philadelphia, 1959.

CHAPTER 3

Tendo Achillis Lengthening

Contracture of the tendo Achillis and consequent shortening of the muscles of the calf is common in association with acquired or congenital talipes equinus and in several paralytic conditions as well.

Simple operative procedures for tendo Achillis lengthening are regularly employed to correct the equinus deformity, but the surgeon must be aware that lengthening is not always helpful. Careful analysis of the nature of calf muscle contracture is essential in any consideration of surgical lengthening of the tendo Achillis. In some instances, the alternative of gastrocnemius recession may be more beneficial (see Chapter 4). Calf muscle contracture is not in itself an indication for lengthening of the tendo Achillis, particularly in patients with cerebral palsy, resistant clubfoot, and paralytic poliomyelitis. In these patients surgical lengthening may actually exacerbate the disability, particularly when calf muscles are weak or the knee has impaired quadriceps control. Contracture of the heel in these instances provides a certain stability that would be lost if the tendo Achillis were lengthened surgically. Gradual lengthening may be accomplished by cast changes or wedging without further weakening of affected muscles.

Otherwise, tendo Achillis lengthening is the treatment of choice when conservative treatment has failed. The procedures shown here are the most commonly employed operative techniques to alleviate plantar flexion. When reoperation is necessary, a Z-plasty must be performed to compensate for previous scarring.

We cannot overemphasize the disadvantages of tendo Achillis lengthening in the face of gastrocnemius equinus. The surgeon must be fully cognizant in performing his pre-op evaluation that an incorrect diagnosis can lead to a useless if not detrimental surgery. It thus behooves the surgeon to evaluate ankle joint dorsiflexion by placing the patient in a prone or supine position with the subtalar joint neutral and the knee extended. With the foot then maximally dorsiflexed, the surgeon must ascertain the availability of motion. If less than 10 degrees of dorsiflexion is present with the knee extended, the existence of a gastrocnemius shortage is plausible. The surgeon must then repeat the examination with the knee in the flexed position. If adequate motion exists in this state a diagnosis of gastrocnemius shortage may be made. However, if dorsiflexion remains unchanged with the knee flexed, a bony ankle block or soleus contracture must be considered. A stress lateral and weight-being lateral radiograph will confirm the surgeon's diagnosis and allow him to perform the procedure which is appropriate to the etiology of the deformity.

Z-plastic Lengthening of the Tendo Achillis

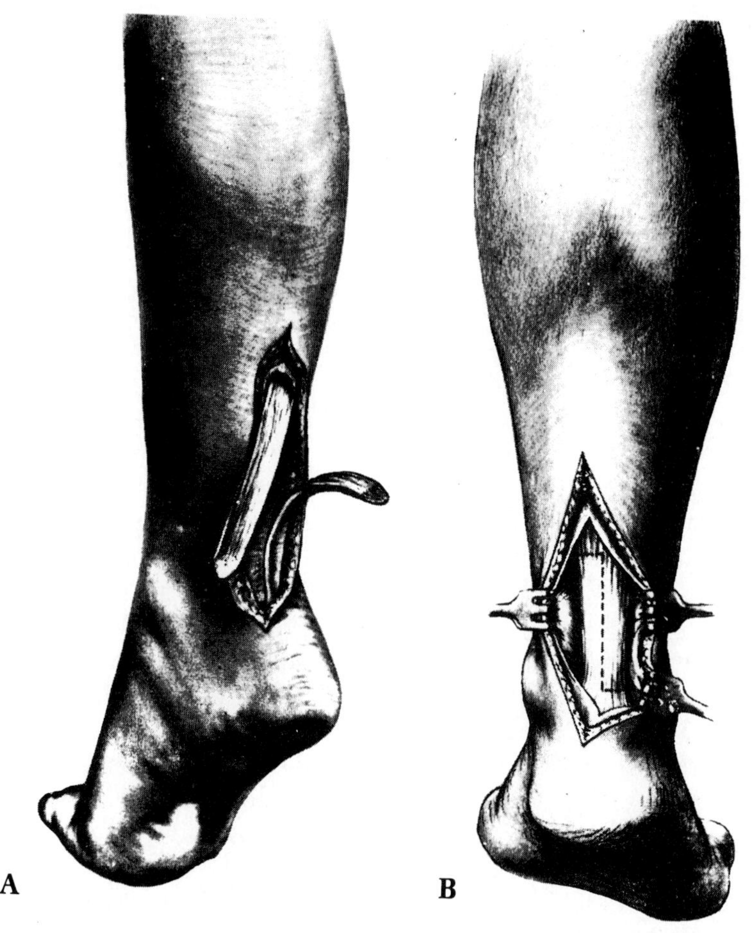

Figure 1. (Reproduced with permission from Crenshaw, A.H. (Ed.): *Campbell's Operative Orthopaedics*, Vol. 2, 5 ed., C.V. Mosby, St. Louis, 1971, p. 1212.)

1. A straight posterior skin incision is made medial to the tendo Achillis.
2. Skin edges are undermined and retracted to expose the sheath of the tendo Achillis.
3. The sheath of the tendo Achillis is incised longitudinally to expose the tendo Achillis, and the small adjacent plantaris longus tendon is cut.
4. A. Lengthening by lateral or frontal plane usually is preferred because the width of the tendon is preserved and the amount of residual cut surface is less.

a. A pointed knife is inserted into the tendon at the proper level and the tendon is split, in the frontal plane, into an anterior half and a posterior half. One half is severed from its base at the lower end and the other at the upper end by transverse incision.
b. This results in two tongue-like halves, the length of which is so calculated that when they are united in the desired position by silk sutures, the tendon will be the desired length.

B. Lengthening by anteroposterior plane is preferred in an equinovarus deformity that leaves the lateral half attached, since the tendo Achillis is often inserted medially and favors recurrence of the rearfoot varus.
a. The tendon is divided longitudinally in its midline, and one half is severed laterally at the upper (proximal) end and the other half medially at the lower (distal) end.
b. This results in two halves, the length of which is so calculated that when they are united in the desired position by silk sutures, the tendon will be the desired length.

5. Tendon sheath is closed with No. 3-0 Dexon® and skin closure is effected with No. 3-0 nylon.
6. The skin over the tendo Achillis just proximal to the heel must be carefully inspected with the foot in the desired position. If the skin is blanched or taut from undue tension, the deformity should only be partially corrected and the foot held in that position when casted to avoid sloughing.
7. Cast is applied from midthigh to toes, with the knee in 30 degree flexion and the ankle in the desired degree of dorsiflexion.
8. After six weeks the cast is removed and passive and active exercises are begun. Walking is allowed in a brace that permits dorsiflexion but prevents plantar flexion.

Hauser Technique[1]

By the Hauser technique, tendo Achillis lengthening is accomplished by means of incomplete tenotomy. The skin incision, exposure of the tendon, and after treatment are the same as for Z-plasty.

The tendon is lengthened by dividing its posterior two-thirds proximally; its medial two-thirds distally. The tendon lengthens as the foot is dorsiflexed.

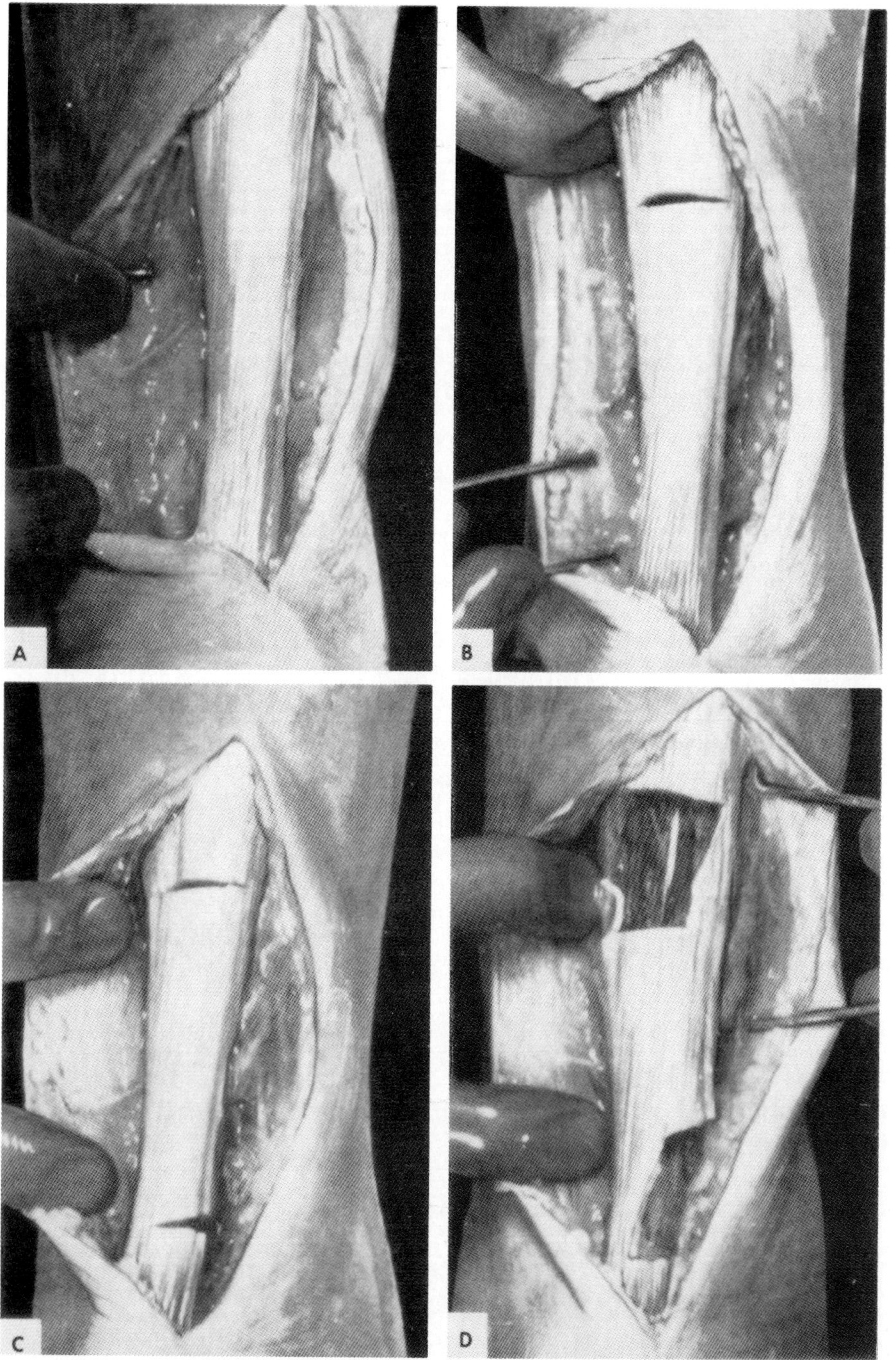

Figure 2. (Reproduced with permission from Cummins, E.J., et al.: The structure of the calcaneal tendon (of Achilles) in relation to orthopedic surgery, *Surg. Gynec. Obstet.*, **83**:107, 1946; courtesy Dr. E.D.W. Hauser.)

White Technique[2]

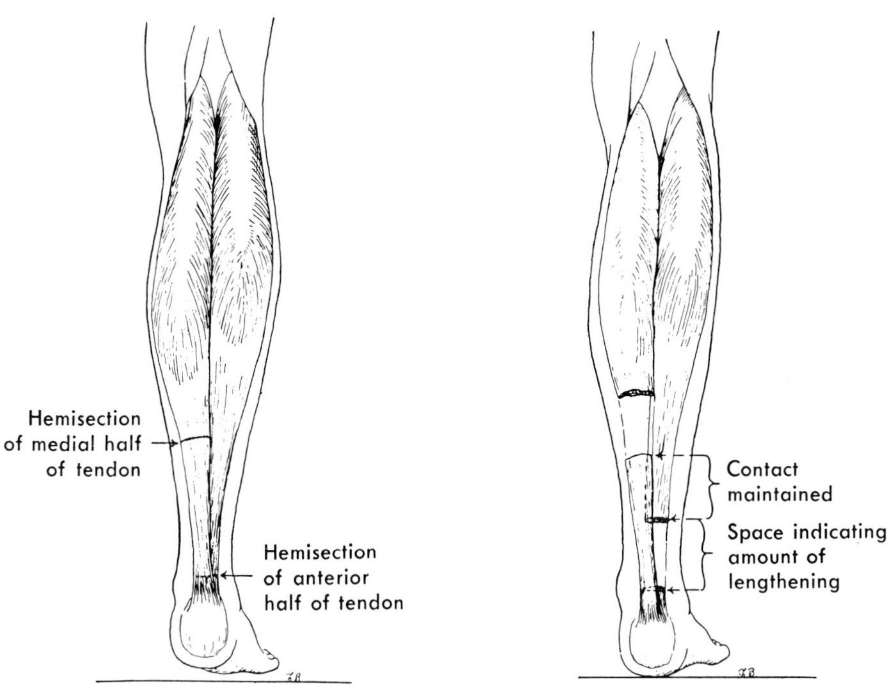

Figure 3. (Reproduced with permission from White, J.W.: Torsion of the Achilles tendon; its surgical significance, *Arch. Surg.*, **46**:784, 1943.)

With the White technique, the skin incision, exposure of the tendon, and after treatment are the same as for Z-plasty. Lengthening is accomplished by incomplete tenotomy.

Divide the anterior two-thirds of the tendon near its insertion. Exert moderate force to dorsiflex the foot, and divide the medial two-thirds of the tendon two to three inches proximally to the site of the first division. Because dorsiflexion of the foot lengthens the tendon, it is not necessary to suture it. From the posterior view the tendon can be observed to rotate 90 degrees, medially to laterally, on its longitudinal axis between its origin and its insertion.

Hibbs Method[3]

With the Hibbs method, the tendon is exposed through the lateral skin incision (A). The medial two-thirds of the tendon is divided proximally, and it is then split longitudinally in the distal direction at the lateral end of the incision. The lateral two-thirds of the tendon is then divided near the point of insertion, and it is split longitudinally in the proximal direction at the medial end of the incision (B). Dorsiflexion of the foot lengthens the tendon while continuity is maintained (C).

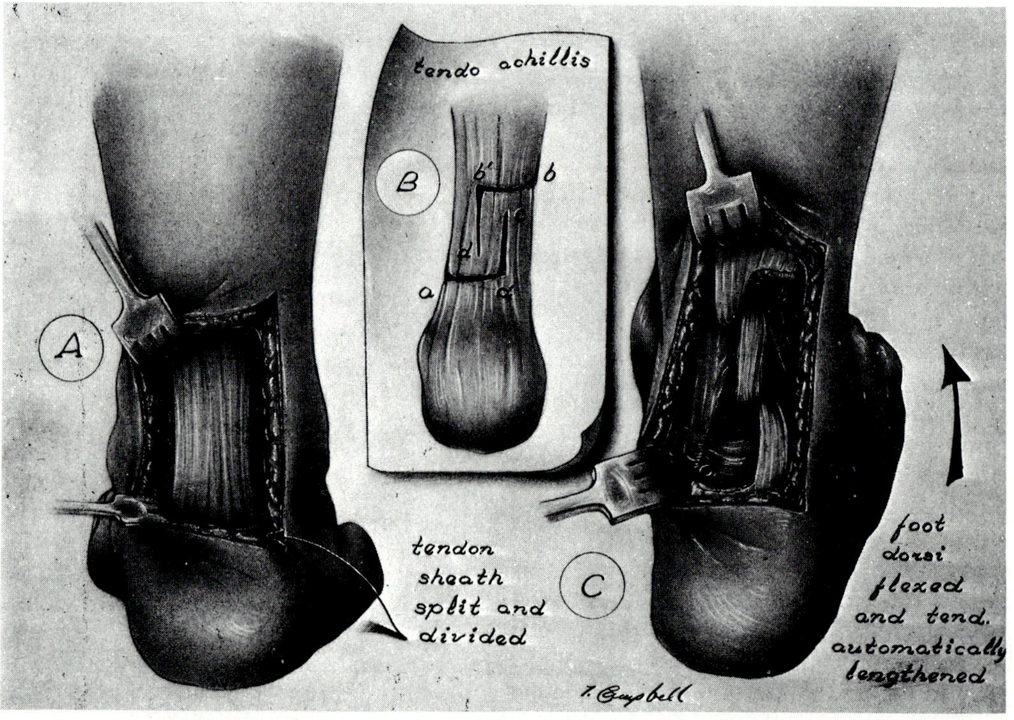

Figure 4. (Reproduced with permission from Giannestras, N.J.: *Foot Disorders: Medical and Surgical Management,* Lea & Febiger, Philadelphia, 1967, p. 154.)

Stewart Technique

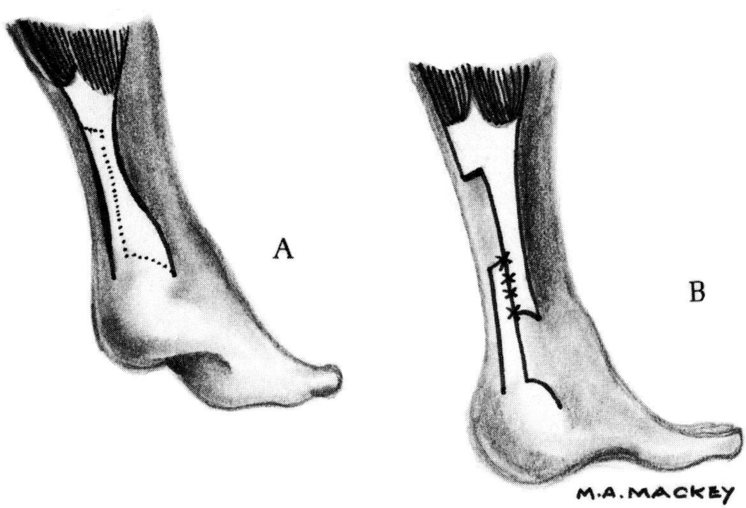

Figure 5a. Stewart technique of tendo Achillis lengthening. (A) Tendon is contracted, its insertion is more medial than normal and extends anteriorly on the medial surface of the calcaneus. Broken line indicates incision in the tendon. (B) Foot is placed in slight dorsiflexion, freeing medial half from the calcaneus, and tendon is sutured in its lengthened position.

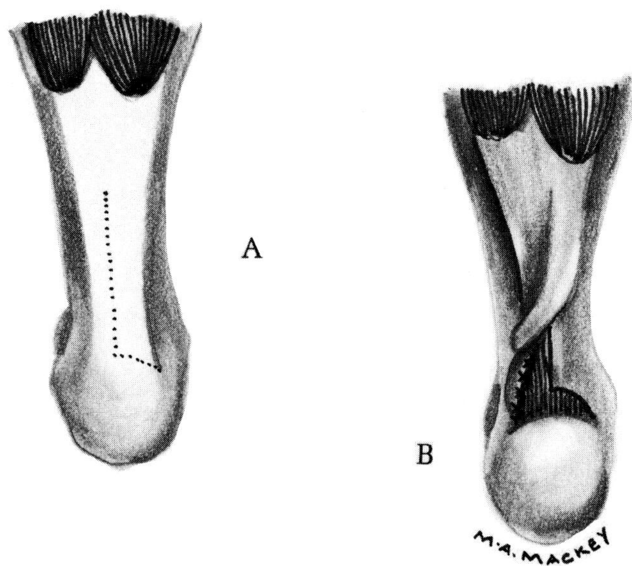

Figure 5b. Stewart technique for transposing tendo Achillis. (A) Tendon is not contracted. Broken line indicates the incision in the tendon. (B) Medial portion is transposed laterally and sutured to the insertion of the lateral portion.

Skin excision, exposure of the tendo Achillis, and after treatment are the same as for Z-plastic lengthening.

1. Z-plastic lengthening in an anteroposterior plane, when the tendon is contracted.
2. When tendon is not contracted:
   a. The tendon is divided longitudinally in its midline and severed medially at the lower, or distal, end.
   b. The medial portion is transposed laterally and sutured to the insertion of the lateral portion.

References

1. Cummins, E.J., et al.: The structure of the calcaneal tendon (of Achilles) in relation to orthopedic surgery, with additional observations on plantaris muscle. *Surg. Gynecol. Obstet.*, **83**:107, 1946.
2. White, J.W.: Torsion of the Achilles tendon, its surgical significance. *Arch. Surg.*, **46**:772, 1943.
3. Giannestras, N.S.: *Foot Disorders*, Lea & Febiger, Philadelphia, 1973, pp. 165–169.

Selected Bibliography

Crenshaw, A.H. (Ed.): *Campbell's Operative Orthopaedics*, Vol. 2, C.V. Mosby, St. Louis, 1971, pp. 1209–1212; 1908–1909.

Frenkenberg, A., Morgan, J., Shane, H.S., and Sgarlato, T.E.: Tendo Achillis lengthening and its effect on foot disorders, *J.A. P.A.*, **65**:849-871, 1975.

Goldstein, L.A., and Dickerson, R.C.: *Atlas of Orthopaedic Surgery*, Vol. 2, C.V. Mosby, St. Louis, 1974, p. 834.

Hibbs, R.A.: Muscle bound feet, *N.Y. Med. J.*, **100**:797–799, 1914, 1974.

Melillo, T.V.: Gastrocnemius equinus, its diagnosis and treatment. *Arch. Pod. Med. and Foot Surg.*, **II**:159–205, 1975.

Sgarlato, T.E., et al.: Tendo Achillis lengthening and its effect on foot disorders, *J.A.P.A.*, **65**:849–871, 1975.

Steindler, A.: *Orthopedic Operations*, Charles C Thomas, Springfield, Ill., 1940, pp. 94–96.

Stewart, S.F.: Club foot, its incidence, causes and treatment. An anatomical physiological study. *J. Bone Jt. Surg.*, **33-A**:577, 1951.

CHAPTER 4

Gastrocnemius Recession

In cases of spastic paralysis with gastrocnemius equinus, the dorsiflexion does not derive from contracture of the tendo Achillis. Therefore, it is inadvisable to employ a surgical technique that involves tendo Achillis lengthening. Lengthening the tendo Achillis would serve only to weaken the soleus muscle, which in combination with the already weak gastrocnemius muscle could cause a hip drop and consequent disequilibrium. In the weakened state the triceps surae cannot resist the reactive force of gravity. Gastrocnemius recession, however, alters nerve impulses from the limb and thereby modifies the extensor reflexes of the triceps surae so that they are able to resist reactive gravitational forces and maintain balance.

Compared with the procedures employed in tendo Achillis lengthening, techniques of gastrocnemius recession have the further advantages of a shorter casting period, reduced convalescence, minimal postoperative balance problems, and better toleration among the older age group.

Anatomically speaking, the gastrocnemius muscle takes origin from the femur and has its insertion into the middle one-third of the posterior aspect of the calcaneus by the Achilles tendon. It is the combined fibers of the gastrocnemius muscle and the soleus muscle which form the Achilles tendon; however, throughout the length and breath of the Achilles tendon the fibers of each tendon are separate and distinct, sharing only a common tendon sheath. As a result the biomechanical functions of the gastrocnemius muscle are unique and the tendon should be considered an entity unto itself. As suggested by Dr. Morton Root and associates, "The term gastrosoleus muscle is a misnomer when considering function."

It is the firm belief of Gray, Basmajian and Sutherland, on the basis of electromyographic studies of muscles of the foot and leg, that the midstance function of the gastrocnemius muscle is to extend the knee. However, as clearly stated by Root et al, the gastrocnemius is not an extensor of the knee but rather functions to prevent hyperextension by exerting flexion tension on the knee. This function is antagonistic to the extensor forces created by the remaining calf muscles, but one must consider that the gastrocnemius muscle takes its origin from the femur. The ability of the gastrocnemius to maintain such flexion thus allows the knee to extend in a smooth manner, prevents hyperextension and lifts the heel to precipitate propulsion. This latter function of the gastrocnemius muscle is quite apparent following gastrocnemius surgery, as the patient exhibits an inability to lift his heel. The patient will subsequently claw his toes and plantar flex the first ray as the extensor digitorium longus and peroneus longus try to assume the impossible task of lifting the heel during propulsion.

Lengthening of Gastrocnemius by Vulpius Technique[1]

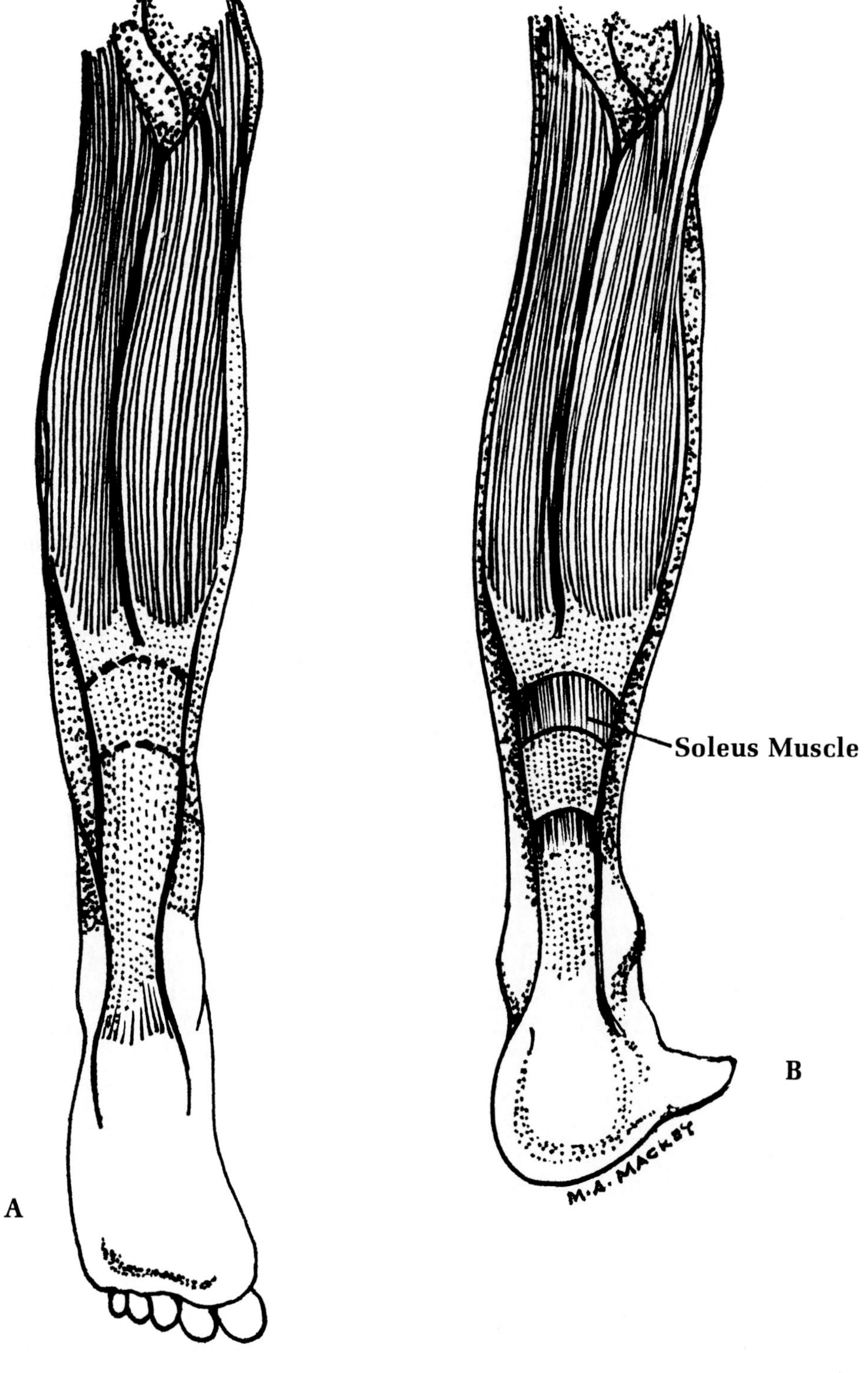

Figure 1. Lengthening of gastrocnemius by Vulpius technique. (A) Broken lines are sites of V-shaped incisions. (B) Foot is forced into slight dorsiflexion separating the segments of the tendon.

1. Posterior longitudinal incision approximately 8 cm long made over middle of calf.
2. Medial sural nerve identified and retracted.
3. Aponeurotic tendon of the gastrocnemius muscle exposed and a V-shaped incision made through it.
4. Ankle forced into slight dorsiflexion to separate the segments of tendon.
5. If the aponeurosis of the soleus is also contracted, divide it, but do not disturb the soleus muscle itself.
6. Cast applied from groin to toes, with knee fully extended and ankle in either slight dorsiflexion or neutral position.
7. *After care*. After six weeks cast is removed, and a single-caliper brace that holds the ankle in the same position is fitted and worn at night until growth is complete.

Lengthening of Gastrocnemius by Baker Technique[2]

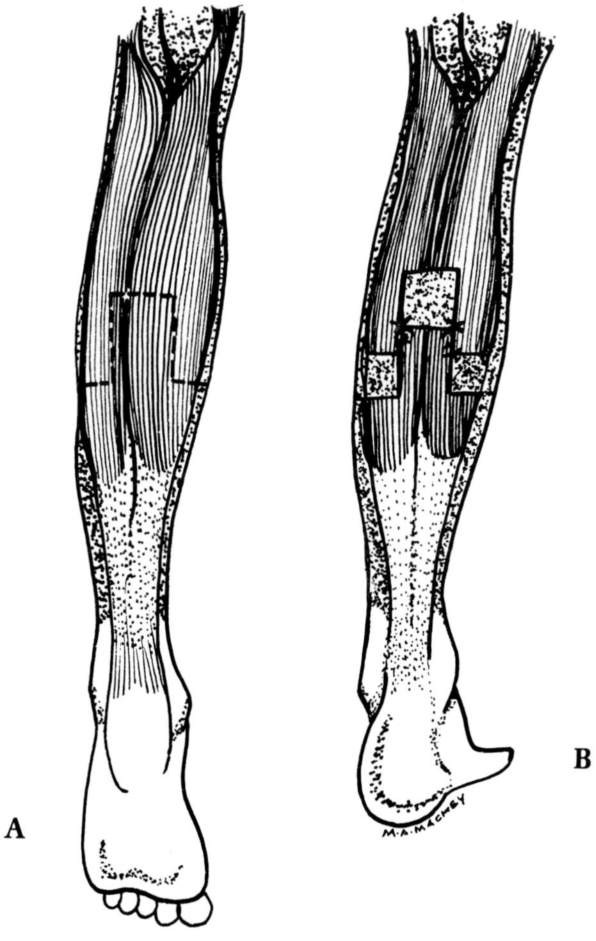

Figure 2. Lengthening of gastrocnemius by Baker technique. (A) Broken line is site of inverted-U incision made through aponeurotic tendon. (B) Foot is placed into slight dorsiflexion and central part of tongue is sutured to the lateral and medial parts with four sutures.

1. Posterior longitudinal incision approximately 8 cm long made over middle of calf.
2. Medial sural nerve identified and retracted.
3. The aponeurotic tendon of the gastrocnemius identified and an inverted-U incision made through the aponeurosis.
4. Middle part of the tongue dissected from the soleus.
5. Central aponeurosis of soleus dissected free to allow full dorsiflexion of the ankle joint.
6. Middle part of tongue sutured in the lengthened position to the lateral and medial parts with four sutures.
7. Fascia and skin closed.

Lengthening of Gastrocnemius by Strayer Technique[3]

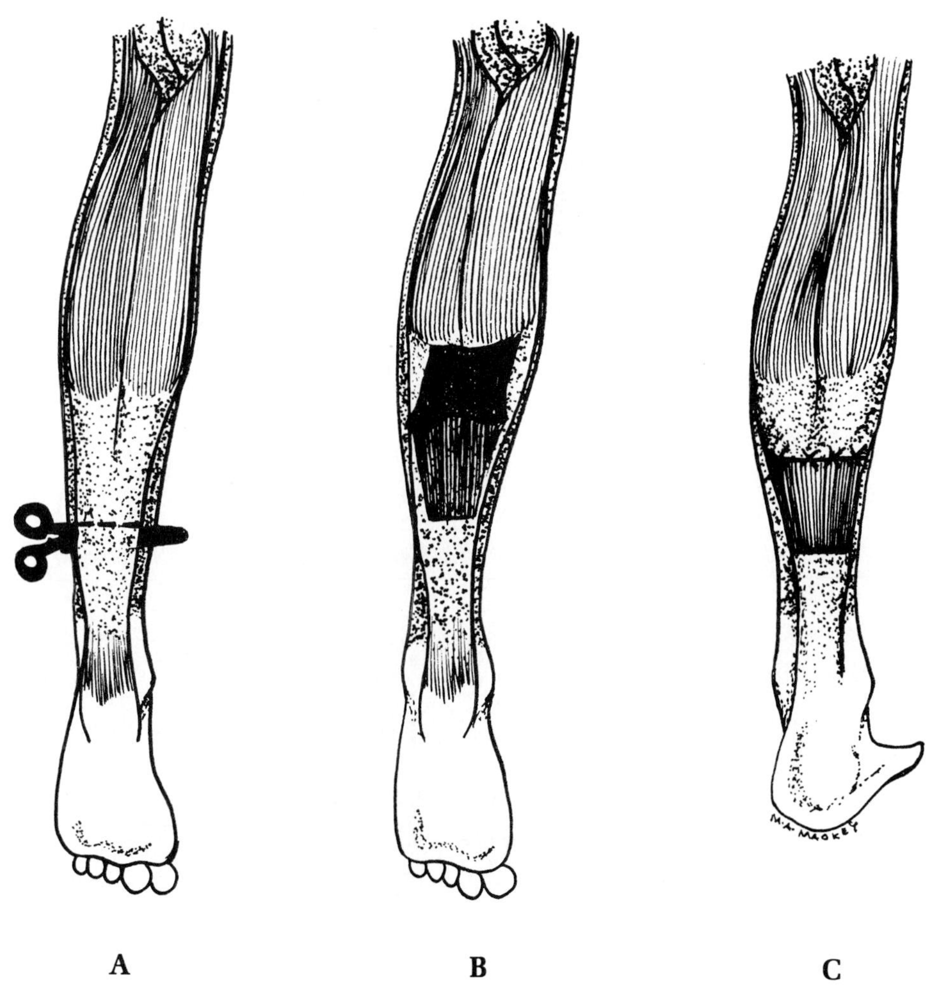

Figure 3. Lengthening of gastrocnemius by Strayer technique. (A) By blunt dissection, gastrocnemius is separated from underlying soleus. Broken line is site of incision into conjoined tendon. (B) Tendon retracted. (C) Foot is forced into slight dorsiflexion and the proximal portion of the apроneurotic tendon is sutured to the underlying soleus.

By this procedure the gastrocnemius is freed completely from the soleus and has a tendency to retract upward, and it may form a useless knot just below the knee. This risk is a distinct disadvantage of the procedure, but its advantage is that it preserves the soleus function for push off in gait.

1. Posterior longitudinal incision approximately 4–6 inches long made over the middle of the calf.
2. Medial sural nerve identified and retracted.
3. Incision deepened through fascia to expose the gastrocnemius muscle.
4. By blunt dissection, gastrocnemius is separated from underlying soleus distally to where its aponeurotic tendon joins the soleus to form the tendo Achillis.
5. Probe inserted deep to the gastrocnemius and its tendon is severed.
6. Foot is dorsiflexed so that a gap ¾–1 inch wide appears between the segments of the severed tendon.
7. The two muscle bellies are then dissected from their medial and lateral attachments to the deep fascia proximally into the popliteal fossa.
8. Gastrocnemius completely separated from soleus by passing a finger from side to side thereby allowing further proximal retraction of the gastrocnemius.
9. Proximal part of the aponeurotic tendon sutured to the underlying soleus with fine interrupted silk sutures at a level at least 1 inch farther proximally than its original attachment.
10. Wound closed with subcuticular catgut or Dexon® suture material.
11. Cast applied from groin to toes with the knee in extension and ankle in a neutral position.
12. *After care.* Intensive exercises are carried out to develop the gluteal muscles. After four weeks the cast is removed and a single-caliper brace that holds the ankle in the same position is fitted and worn at night until growth is complete and the muscles have regained their tone.

References

1. Crenshaw, A.H. (Ed.): *Campbell's Operative Orthopaedics*, Vol. 2, C.V. Mosby, St. Louis, 1971, pp. 1698–1699.
2. Baker, L.D.: *J. Bone Jt. Surg.*, **38-A**:318, 1956.
3. Strayer, L.M., Jr.: *J. Bone Surg.*, **32-A**:671, 1950.

Selected Bibliography

McGlamry, E.D. (Ed.): *Reconstructive Surgery of the Foot and Leg*, Intercontinental Medical Book Corporation, New York, 1974, pp. 280–282.

Root, M.L., Orien, W.P., and Weed, J.H.: *Normal and Abnormal Function of the Foot*, Clinical Biomechanical Corporation, Los Angeles, 1978.

Tachdjian, M.O.: *Pediatric Orthopaedics*, Vol. 2, W.B. Saunders, Philadelphia, 1972, pp. 794–798.

CHAPTER 5

Tendo Achillis Repair

Diagnosis of a tendo Achillis rupture becomes more difficult with time. A newly ruptured tendo Achillis usually exhibits a gap in the tendon, however the later formation of a hemotoma with subsequent edema into the tendon sheath can cause the gap to be filled and the diagnosis to be missed.

As a result, an adequate examination must place the patient in a prone position with his feet extending over the table's edge. The surgeon must then squeeze the calf muscles in the middle one-third below the place of widest girth. If no plantar movement exists one must conclude that a rupture of the Achilles tendon exists. An individual will also exhibit an excessive range of dorsiflexion, much greater than would be achieved by tendo Achillis lengthening alone.

Surgical repair of a ruptured tendo Achillis is difficult to accomplish without residual effects, including muscle weakness and adhesions. In most cases rupture results in longitudinal tearing of the tendon tissue into irregular strips either at the musculotendinous junction or at the point of insertion into the calcaneus—the two most common sites of rupture.

Various techniques for surgical repair of a ruptured tendo Achillis have been developed, and timing of the diagnosis is a critical factor in selection of the correct procedure for repair.

For diagnostic and surgical purposes it is important to realize that in middle-aged people rupture commonly occurs at the point of insertion of the tendon into the calcaneus, whereas in younger patients it generally occurs near the musculotendinous junction. If a distal diagnosis is made within ten days of the injury, the Lynn technique is ideal. Because it involves reinforcing the tendo Achillis with the plantaris tendon, this method must be performed early, before the plantaris tendon becomes incorporated into the scar tissue.

For a proximal rupture McLaughlin's technique is preferred, and it is particularly helpful in the case of a late repair. The procedure involves excision of the frayed or torn ends of the tendon, a process that may shorten the tendon by as much as 10 cm. A defect even that large, however, can be compensated for by increasing the flexure of the ankle and the knee. To avoid excessive pull of the triceps surae, surgical repair is accomplished with removable wire sutures.

Other methods developed by Goldstein and Dickerson, by Bosworth, and by Lindholm involve reinforcement of the torn tendon with living fascia grafts from the posterior surface of the gastrocnemius muscle. The Bosworth procedure is used for late repair of a rupture.

Lynn Technique

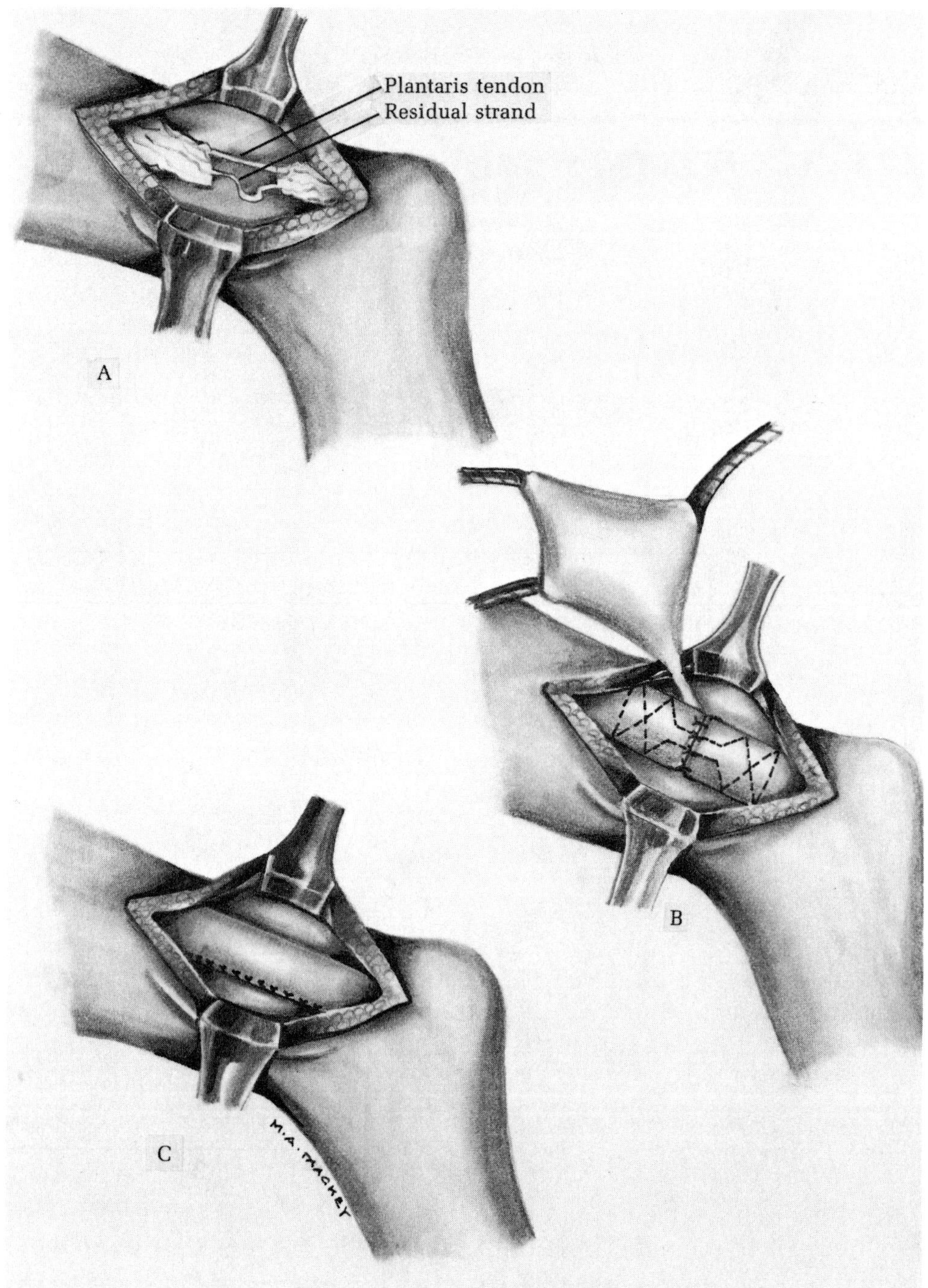

Figure 1a. Lynn technique for repair of fresh rupture of tendo Achillis. (A) Torn ends of fresh rupture of tendo Achillis and plantaris tendon are intact. (B) Tendon has been repaired. The tendon of the plantaris has been freed from its distal attachment and fanned out into a membrane. (C) Repair is complete. The fanned-out tendon of the plantaris is wrapped around the tendo Achillis and sutured to it by the edges.

I. Fresh Rupture

1. An incision 5–7 inches long is made parallel to the medial border of the tendo Achillis.
2. The tendon sheath is opened in the midline and with the foot held in 20 degrees plantar flexion, and without excising the irregular edges, the ends of the tendo Achillis are sutured with fine chromic catgut.
3. If the plantaris tendon is intact, its insertion at the calcaneus is divided and the tendon is fanned out to form a membrane.
4. Place the membrane over the repair of the tendo Achillis and suture it in place with interrupted sutures. When possible, cover the tendo Achillis for 1 inch both proximally and distally to the repair.
5. If the plantaris tendon is also ruptured, dissect it free from the tendo Achillis for several inches and divide it through a small second incision in the middle of the calf. The tendon is then pulled distally into the first incision and fanned out as a free graft, and the repair is covered.
6. The sheath of the tendo Achillis is closed as far distally as possible without tension.
7. Skin closure is effected in the usual manner.

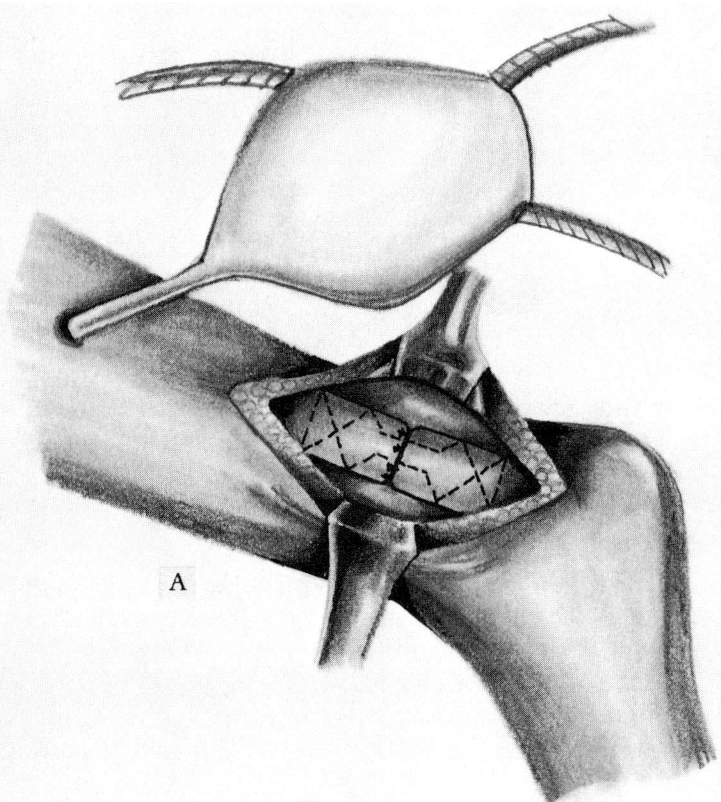

Figure 1b. Lynn technique for repair of a ten-day-old rupture of the tendo Achillis. (A) Plantaris tendon is dissected free from the tendo Achillis and brought out through an incision in the calf and fanned out into a membrane. Tendon has been repaired. *(Continued on next page).*

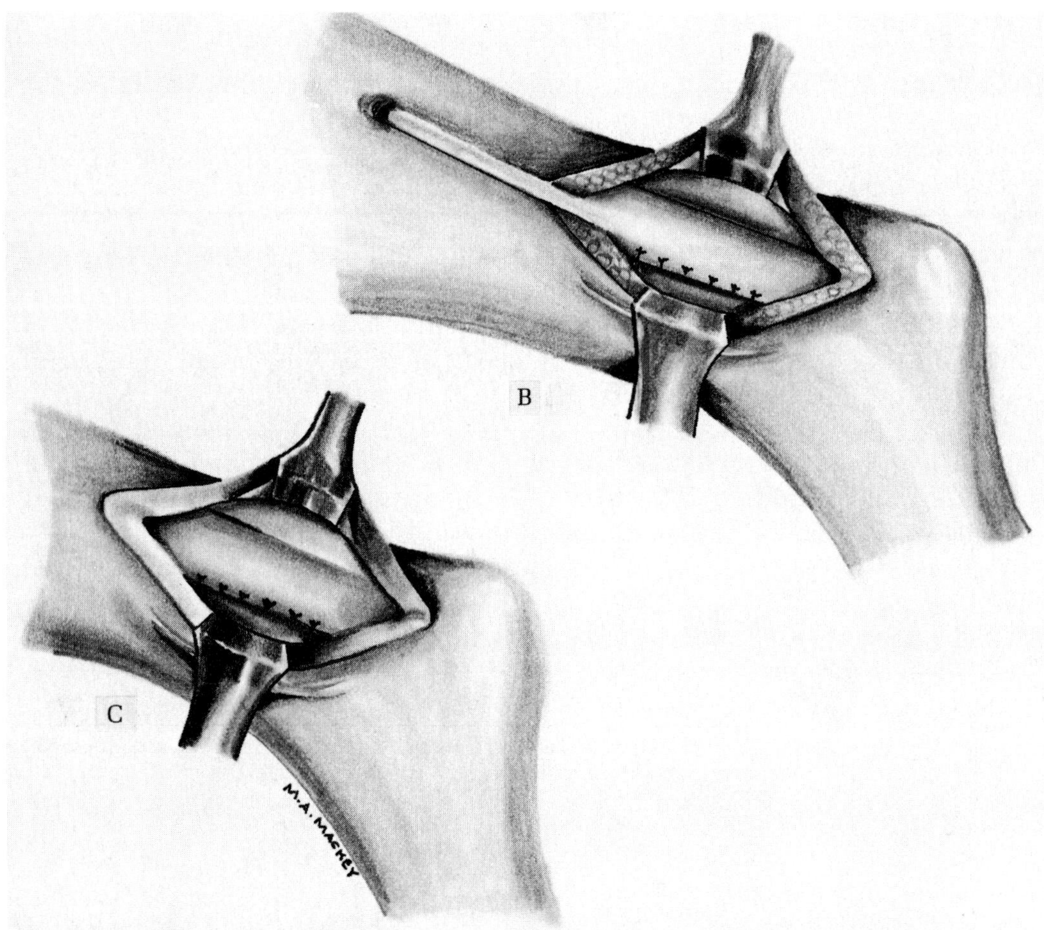

Figure 1b (continued). Lynn technique for repair of a ten-day-old rupture of the tendo Achillis. (B) The fanned-out tendon of the plantaris is brought into the wound and wrapped around the tendo Achillis and sutured to it by the edges. (C) Redundant portion discarded and repair complete.

II. Ten-day-old Rupture

1. Surgical approach to tendon is same as for fresh rupture.
2. Tendon is bridged with a slender bit of fibrous tissue which is excised, and the ends of the tendo Achillis are sutured together.
3. The plantaris tendon is dissected free from the tendo Achillis for several inches along its length and is divided through a small second incision in the middle of the calf.
4. The tendon is then pulled distally into the first incision and fanned out as a free graft, and the repair is covered.
5. The sheath of the tendo Achillis is closed as far distally as possible without tension, and the redundant portion is discarded.
6. Skin closure is effected in the usual manner.

III. Casting

1. The skin over the tendo Achillis just proximal to the heel must be carefully inspected with the foot in the desired position. If the skin is blanched or taut from undue tension, the foot should be maintained in equinus to relieve tension on the sutures and avoid sloughing.
2. A long leg cast is applied with the foot in equinus and the knee in flexion.

IV. After Care

1. Cast is removed after six weeks, and a short leg cast is then applied with the foot in slight equinus.
2. The patient gradually resumes walking with partial weight-bearing on crutches during the next two weeks; the walking is allowed without crutches.
3. After four to six more weeks, the cast is removed and walking and weight-bearing are gradually resumed in a reverse 90 degree ankle-stop brace that is worn for three months.

McLaughlin's Technique[1]

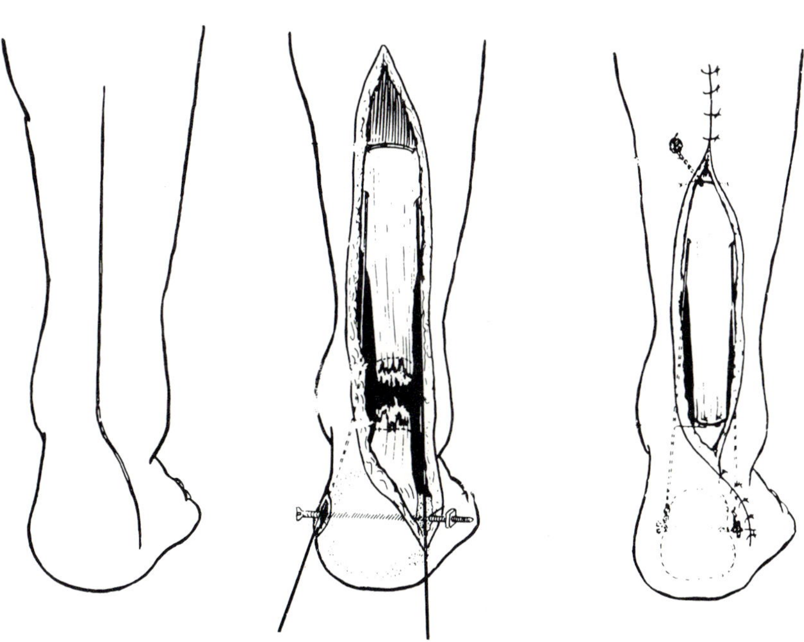

Figure 2. Repair of ruptured tendo Achillis by removable suture. (Reproduced with permission from Giannestras, N.J.: *Foot Disorders: Medical and Surgical Management,* Lea & Febiger, Philadelphia, 1967, p. 425.)

1. A midline incision is made which curves laterally in its distal portion to avoid shoe pressure on the scar.
2. The frayed and fragile tendon edges are trimmed back to reasonably healthy tissue.
3. A drill hole is made medially to laterally through the calcaneus, and a stab wound is made at its point of emergence.
4. A long screw is passed through the drill hole in the calcaneus.
5. A wire suture is inserted into the proximal tendon fragment, which is then pulled into position by the two ends of the wire suture which are fastened to the projecting ends of the screw.
6. With retraction thus counteracted, the trimmed tendon ends are sutured together.
7. The superfluous portion of the screw is cut free and removed.
8. A twisted wire with a split lead shot (for palpable localization of the mattress suture) is attached to the proximal portion of the wire suture.
9. A plaster of Paris cast is applied as in the Lynn Technique.
10. *After care.* Immobilization is maintained for eight weeks, after which the screw, washer, and wire sutures are removed. Active weight-bearing is then begun.

Goldstein and Dickerson Technique[2]

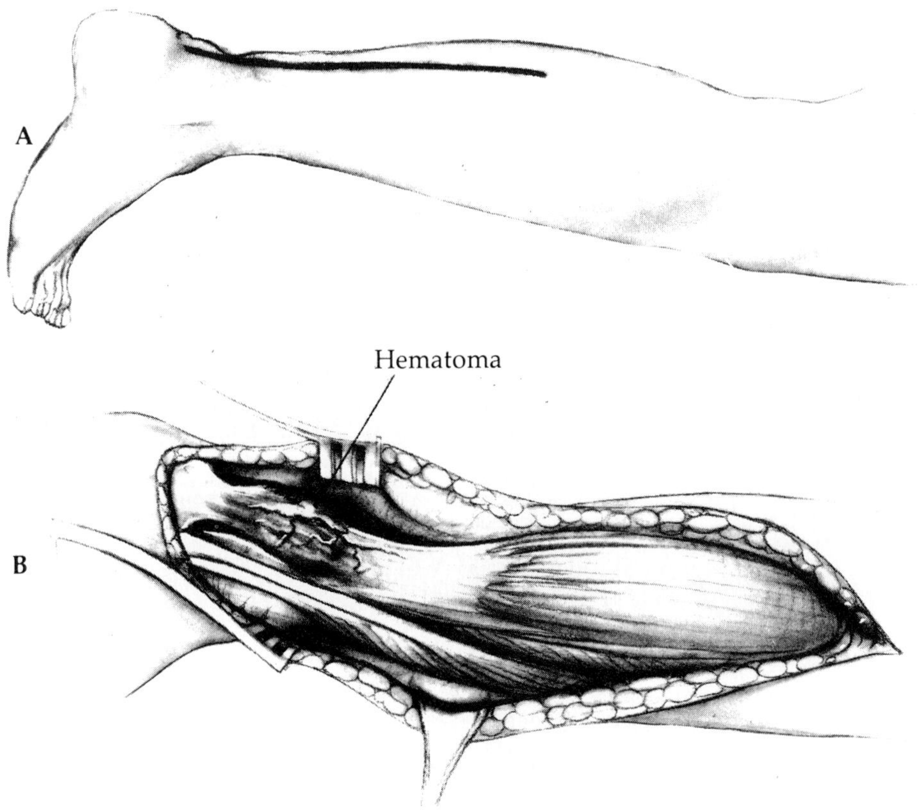

Figure 3. Repair of ruptured Achilles tendon. (Reproduced with permission from Goldstein, L. A., and Dickerson, R.C.: *Atlas of Orthopaedic Surgery*, Vol. 2, C.V. Mosby, St. Louis, 1974, pp. 843–847.)

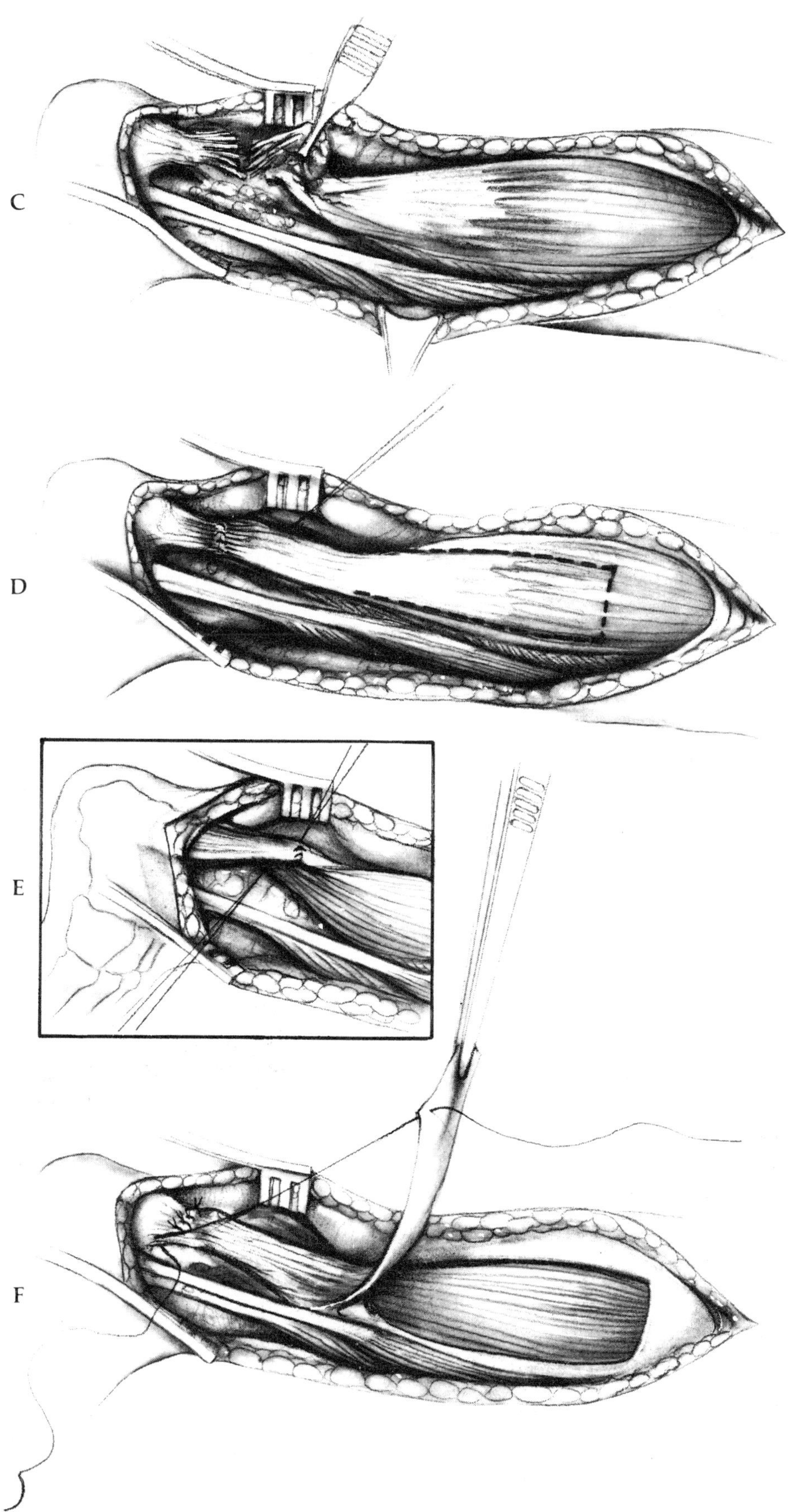
C
D
E
F

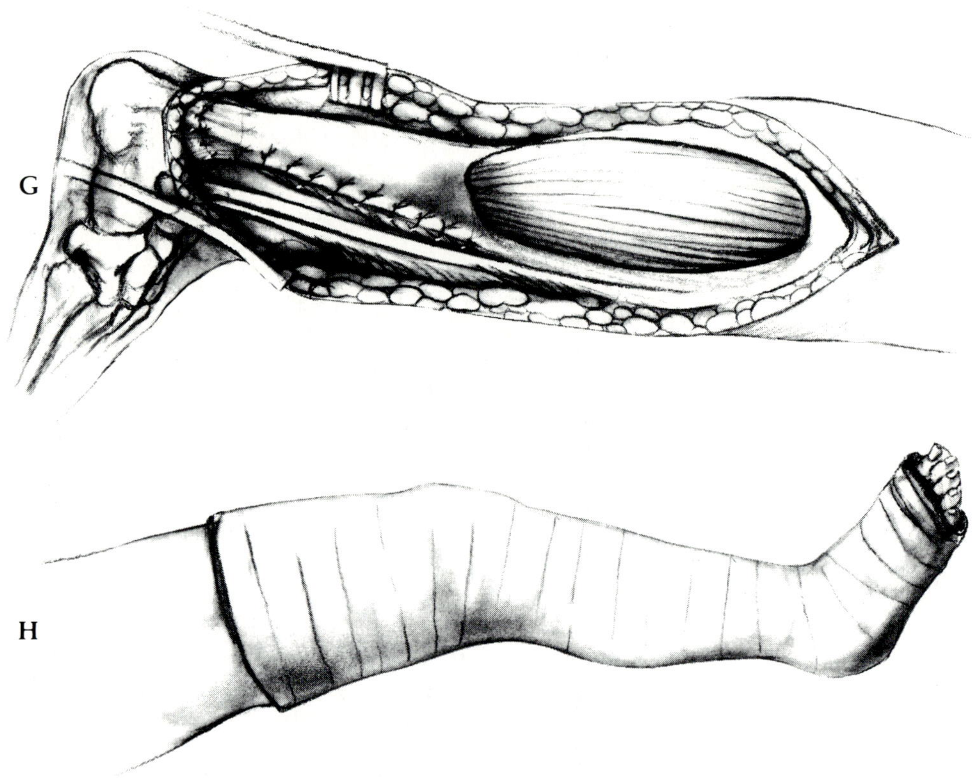

Figure 3 (continued). Repair of ruptured Achilles tendon. (Reproduced with permission from Goldstein, L.A., and Dickerson, R.C.: *Atlas of Orthopaedic Surgery*, Vol. 2, C.V. Mosby, St. Louis, 1974, pp. 843–847.)

1. A posterior longitudinal incision is made from the midcalf to the level of the posterior margin of the calcaneal tuberosity.
2. When the injury has been recent, the location of the rupture will be marked by a subcutaneous hematoma (B). The ends of the ruptured tendon are usually shredded and irregular (C). The adjacent plantaris tendon, if present, may remain intact.
3. The divided ends of the ruptured tendo Achillis are reapproximated with interrupted mattress sutures circumferentially with the foot in 5–10 degrees plantar flexion (D,E).
4. A long tongue of fascia overlying the posterior surface of the gastrocnemius is then outlined in such a manner that its base (distally) can remain intact and it can be reversed back over the initial end-to-end suturing of the ruptured tendo Achillis (F).
5. The fascia is sutured on both sides of the end-to-end suturing of the ruptured tendon with multiple sutures to provide supplemental reinforcement of the direct end-to-end repair of the ruptured tendo Achillis (G).
6. The surgically created defect where the fascia has been removed over the gastrocnemius muscle may be left open or partially closed without tension or constriction of the underlying posterior calf muscles.
7. Closure is effected in the usual manner.

8. A long leg cast is applied extending from the midthigh to the toes, with the ankle in 5–10 degrees plantar flexion (H).
9. *After care.* After six weeks, a short leg walking cast or a brace with an ankle stop is applied to prevent passive dorsiflexion of the ankle above neutral for an additional six weeks. Weight-bearing activities are then gradually resumed without external protection, but activities that involve forceful or potential sudden stress on the repaired tendon should be avoided for at least four months postoperatively.

Lindholm Procedure[3,4]

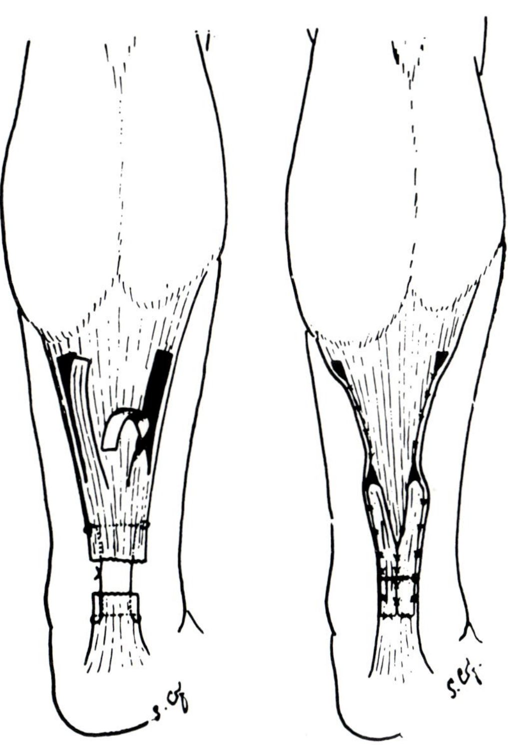

Figure 4. Technique for repairing ruptures of tendo calcaneus. (Reproduced with permission from Lindholm, Å.: A new method of operation in subcutaneous rupture of the Achilles tendon, *Acta Chir. Scand.*, **117**:261, 1959.)

1. A posterior curvilinear incision is made from the midcalf to the calcaneus.
2. The deep fascia is incised in the midline to expose the tendon rupture.
3. The ragged ends of the tendon are debrided and apposed with a box-type mattress suture of heavy silk or wire, and with fine interrupted sutures.
4. From the proximal tendon and gastrocnemius aponeurosis, two flaps are fashioned, each approximately 1 cm wide and 7–8 cm long.
5. These flaps are left attached at a point 3 cm proximal to the site of rupture, and each flap is twisted 180 degrees on itself so that its smooth external surface lies next to the subcutaneous tissues as it is turned distally over the rupture.

6. Each flap is sutured to the distal stump of the tendon and to the other flap, completely covering the site of the rupture.
7. Wound is closed in the usual manner.
8. Casting and after care are the same as for the Lynn procedure.

Bosworth Procedure[5]

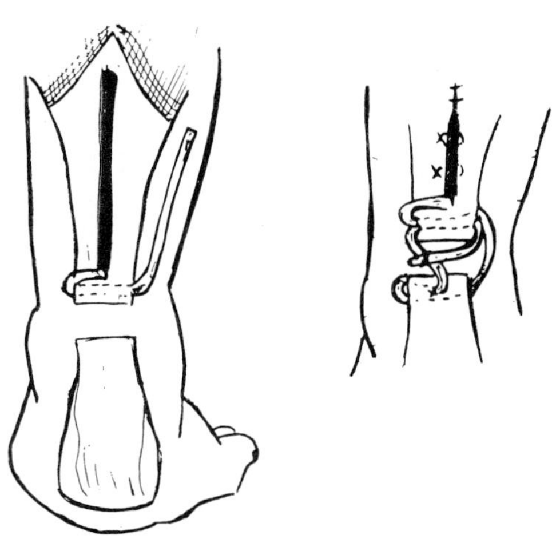

Figure 5. (Reproduced with permission from Kitting, R.W.: Rupture of the Achilles Tendon and Related Considerations. In E.D. McGlamry (Ed.): *Reconstructive Surgery of the Foot and Leg,* Symposia Specialists, Inc., Miami, Fl., 1974, pp. 290–291.)

1. Expose the ruptured tendon by a posterior longitudinal midline incision from the calcaneus to the proximal one-third of the calf.
2. Excise scar tissue from ruptured ends.
3. Free from the median raphe of the gastrocnemius muscle a strip of tendon ½ inch wide and approximately 7 inches long. Leave this strip attached just proximal to the rupture site.
4. Turn the strip down distally and pass it transversely through the proximal tendon and secure it there with chromic catgut.
5. Pass the strip distally and transversely through the distal end of the tendon.
6. Then again pass the tendon through the distal end from anterior to posterior, while holding the knee at 90 degrees and the ankle in plantar flexion. Draw the tendon strip taut and anchor with chromic catgut.
7. Once again, bring the strip proximally and pass it transversely through the proximal end of the tendon.
8. Finally, carry the strip distally and secure it upon itself.
9. Closure is effected in the usual manner.
10. Casting and after care are as described for the Lynn technique.

References

1. Giannestras, N.J.: *Foot Disorders*, Lea & Febiger, Philadelphia, 1967, pp. 424, 428.
2. Goldstein, L.A., and Dickerson, R.C.: *Atlas of Orthopaedic Surgery*, Vol. 2, C.V. Mosby, St. Louis, 1974, pp. 842–847.
3. Lindholm, A.: A new method of operation in subcutaneous rupture of the Achilles tendon. *Acta Chir. Scand.* **117**:261, 1959.
4. Crenshaw, A.H. (Ed.): *Campbell's Operative Orthopaedics*, Vol. 2, C.V. Mosby, St. Louis, 1971, pp. 1465–1469.
5. Kitting, R.W.: Rupture of the Achilles tendon and related considerations. In McGlamry, E.D. (Ed.): *Reconstructive Surgery of the Foot and Leg*, Intercontinental Medical Book Corporation, New York, 1974.

Selected Bibliography

Inman, V.T. (Ed.): *DuVries' Surgery of the Foot*, C.V. Mosby, St. Louis, 1973, p. 198.

Lynn, R.A.: Repair of torn Achilles tendon using the plantaris tendon as a reinforcing membrane, *J. Bone Jt. Surg.*, **48-A**:268, 1966.

McLaughlin, H.L.: *Trauma*, W.B. Saunders, Philadelphia, 1959, p. 367.

CHAPTER 6

Triple Arthrodesis

In several conditions of varying etiologies, painless weight-bearing on the foot becomes impossible. In many such cases arthrodesis, or fusion, of one or more joints of the foot is the treatment of choice. Although fusion prohibits function, the disabling effects of arthrodesis are offset by restoration of the stabilizing function of the foot. The effects of tuberculous lesions, infections, paralytic conditions, arthritis, or trauma may affect the lower limb and foot to the degree that arthrodesis becomes necessary. There are three major types of arthrodesis and numerous surgical techniques. The choice of arthrodesis is dictated by the nature of the defect, the disease state involved, the age of the patient, and the local condition of the bone tissue to be subjected to fusion.

Types of Arthrodesis

1. Intra-articular fusion: exposure of the joint through capsular incision and removal of articular cartilage, subchondral bone, and diseased tissue, with direct approximation of the cancellous bone surfaces.
2. Extra-articular fusion: avoids exposure of the joint surfaces and bridges the joint, usually with bone grafts.
3. Combination: used primarily to obtain a greater area of bone contact and to add strength to the arthrodesis.

The choice of approach to the individual case is also determined by the purpose of any arthrodesis—to join the raw surfaces of bony tissues so that fusion is firm and complete. To accomplish this goal, the adjacent structures must be maintained in close contact so that they will unite. Compression is a useful method that can be accomplished by numerous mechanical techniques and devices—generally both internally and externally applied. Screws, pins, or plates may be used internally to maintain close approximation of the bone surfaces to be fused, and external pressure may be applied by casting until bone regrowth is complete.

Three major joints, the talocalcaneal, the talonavicular, and the calcaneocuboid, work together to control lateral and medial stability of the foot. Because of the interaction of these joints, the need for arthrodesis of one generally means fusion of the other two as well. The most common technique for triple arthrodesis of the foot is the Ryerson procedure, first introduced in 1923. Before that time, Hoke, Davis, and Dunn all had performed surgical stabilization of the subtalar, talonavicular, and cuboid joints; Ryerson, however, identified the calcaneocuboid joint as an essential component of medial and lateral motion. By including this joint in the arthrodesis procedure, it is possible to compensate fully for numerous deformities resulting from paralytic disease, trauma, infection, arthritis, and congenital deformation.

In treating patients with paralytic disease, when a triple arthrodesis is performed, the muscles of the foot must be reinserted in such a way that pull on the bones of the foot will be in balance. Unless this is accomplished, misdirected muscle forces of inversion, eversion, plantar flexion, and dorsiflexion will have a negative structural effect that may in itself cause new deformity or relapse.

In any patient undergoing triple arthrodesis, it is important to note the relation of the talus to the ankle mortise. Without medial and lateral stability of the talus, an arthrodesis is doomed to failure. Stress imposed by a medially or laterally tipping talus will impose stress on the ankle joint during walking; over time the stress may lead to relapse, deformity, or traumatic arthritis of the ankle joint. In patients with triple arthrodesis, ankle fusion is to be avoided (see Chapter 14).

In children who require triple arthrodesis, it is important to defer the operation until the bones have ossified—approximately age 10.

Techniques involving wedge removal and reshaping of the talus have been developed to correct specific deformities, including foot varus, foot valgus, and incorrect subtalar alignment. Hoke's triple arthrodesis involves repositioning a talar graft. This technique can be applied to correct any type of foot deformity as long as the talar graft is properly positioned. In cases of combined equinovarus, calcaneovalgus, equinovalgus, and calcaneovarus, the graft must be placed between the navicular and the talus so that the foot cannot move into its deformed position. For this modification of Hoke's technique, the foot is moved far posteriorly on the talus so that balance can be maintained.

Ryerson Triple Arthrodesis[1,2]

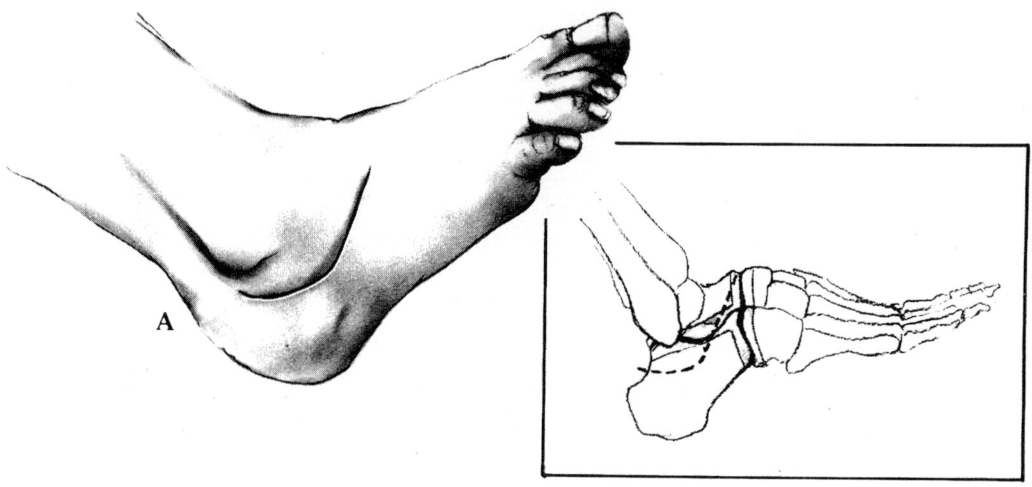

Figure 1a. (Reproduced with permission from Goldstein, L.A., and Dickerson, R.C.: *Atlas of Orthopaedic Surgery*, Vol. 2, C.V. Mosby, St. Louis, 1974, pp. 895, 897.)

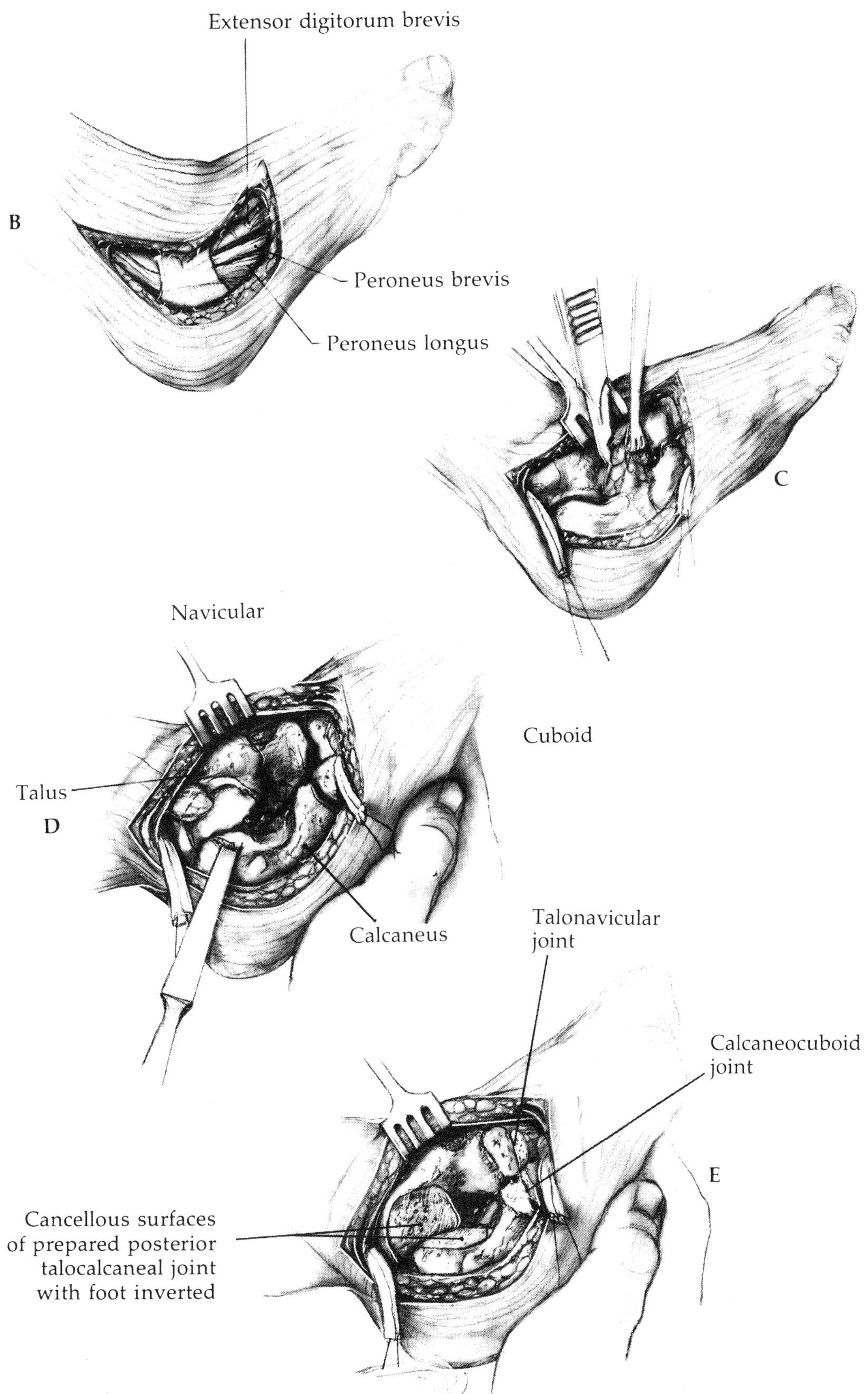
Extensor digitorum brevis
B
Peroneus brevis
Peroneus longus
C
Navicular
Cuboid
Talus
D
Calcaneus
Talonavicular joint
Calcaneocuboid joint
E
Cancellous surfaces of prepared posterior talocalcaneal joint with foot inverted

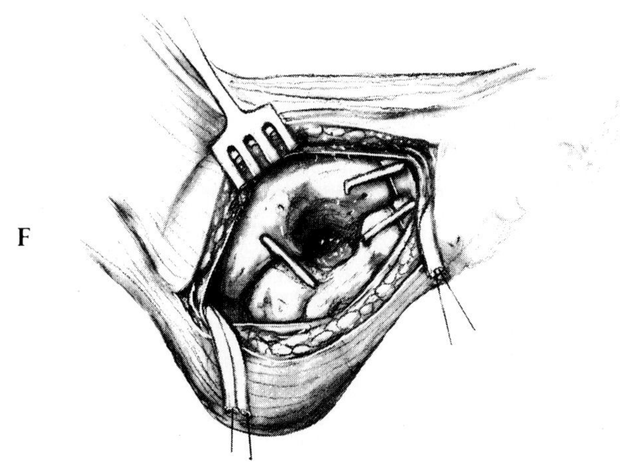

Figure 1a (continued). (Reproduced with permission from Goldstein, L.A., and Dickerson, R.C.: *Atlas of Orthopaedic Surgery*, Vol. 2, C.V. Mosby, St. Louis, 1974, pp. 895, 897.)

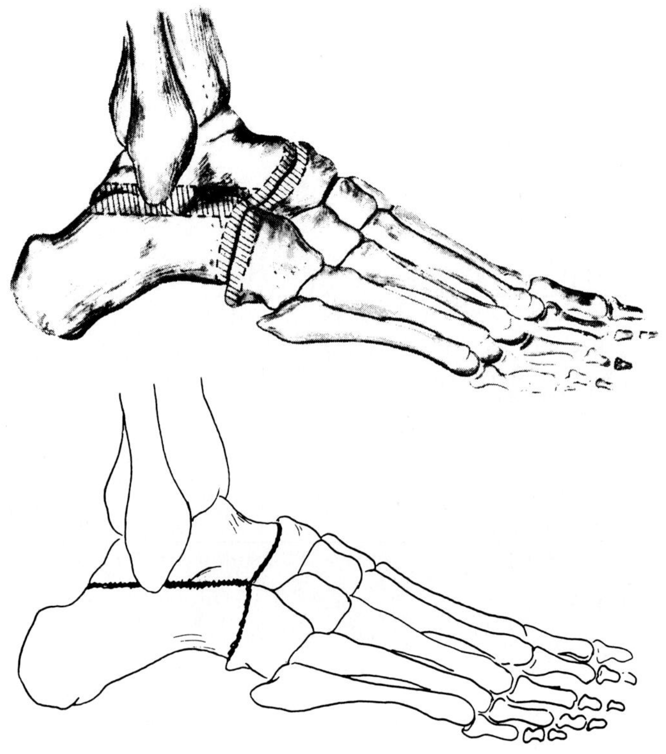

Figure 1b. (Reproduced with permission from Steindler, A.: *Orthopaedic Operations: Indications, Technique, and End Results*, Charles C Thomas, Springfield, Ill., 1940, p. 329.)

Technique

1. May be done with one straight incision centered over the sinus tarsi extended from the peroneus brevis anteriorly toward the head of the talus and ending at the lateral border of the extensor tendons, or by two incisions medially and laterally to minimize the trauma of skin retraction. The first (Ollier) incision on the lateral surface begins at the talonavicular joint and extends downward and backward to end 1 inch below and in back of the lateral malleolus. A second incision is made medially, starting at the base of the first metatarsal and extended posteriorly to just below the tip of the medial malleolus.
2. The sheath of the peroneal tendons is opened and the tendons are retracted plantarly.
3. The origin of the extensor brevis digitorum muscle is dissected from the bone and retracted toward the toes, exposing the sinus tarsi.
4. The fat and fibrous tissue of the sinus tarsi is excised.
5. The calcaneocuboid joint capsule is incised and stripped away from the articular margins by subperiosteal dissection.
6. The anterior articular process of the calcaneus is removed with an osteotome parallel to the base of the sinus tarsi. This bone is saved to be used as a bone graft.
7. The articular surfaces of the calcaneocuboid joint are then removed parallel to each other.
8. The capsule of the subtalar joint is stripped subperiosteally from the sinus tarsi posteriorly to the posterior aspect of the joint, and the opposing surfaces of the subtalar joint are removed from the talus and the calcaneus with a sharp osteotome. This joint curves upward and backward, and the osteotome must follow the configuration of the joint. The cut surfaces may adhere to the posterior and medial joint capsule but can be pried loose by placing a curette behind them and pulling forward and laterally.
9. The talonavicular joint is incised, and the joint surfaces of the talus and navicular are removed.
10. The cut joint surfaces are then fitted together accurately with the foot in normal alignment. The position of the heel is important. It should be in a neutral or slight valgus position, but never in a varus position.
11. The bone chips that have been removed are packed around the sinus tarsi and the talonavicular area (most likely site of pseudoarthrodesis).
12. Wound is closed by suturing the ligaments with a few interrupted sutures.
13. The extensor brevis digitorium is then replaced and sutured.
14. Subcutaneous sutures are usually not necessary and skin is closed.
15. If desired, the tarsus may be held in the correct position by transfixing the joints with Kirschner wires (Caldwell modification), which are removed later.
16. A well-padded plaster cast is applied from the tip of the toes to the midthigh. This is most easily done by hanging the leg over the edge of the operating table and applying the cast from the toes to just below the knee. The alignment of the foot with the leg can be more easily determined with the leg in this position, and the cast can be molded more accurately. When the cast is set, the cast is extended above the partially flexed knee to midthigh.

Postoperative Care

Following the operation, the leg is elevated and may be supported by a sling suspended from an overhead frame. The circulation in the toes must be checked hourly for the first 48 hours, since considerable swelling can occur and circulation may fail quickly, demanding immediate opening of the cast. Adequate analgesics must be given since this is one of the most painful of orthopedic operations. The leg should remain elevated for seven to ten days until the swelling has completely subsided. The patient may then be ambulatory on crutches. After ten to fourteen days the patient is prepared for general anesthesia and the cast is removed. If alignment is satisfactory both clinically and by x-ray, a snug boot cast is applied. Otherwise the foot is manipulated with the patient under general anesthesia for proper alignment. A snug boot cast is then applied and this cast is worn for four weeks while the patient remains on crutches. A walking cast is applied at this time and weight-bearing is gradually resumed. At the end of six more weeks, the cast is removed and x-rays are taken. If fusion is not complete, cast immobilization must continue. If union is present, the foot and leg are wrapped with an ace bandage, and a shoe with a rigid extended counter is worn. Active exercise and gentle massage are started to mobilize the remaining intact joints. Moderate swelling can be anticipated for several weeks and there may be some discomfort in the ankle and forefoot joints until they are fully mobilized.

Triple Arthrodesis with Bone Wedge Removal[3]

I. Reconstruction for valgus deformity

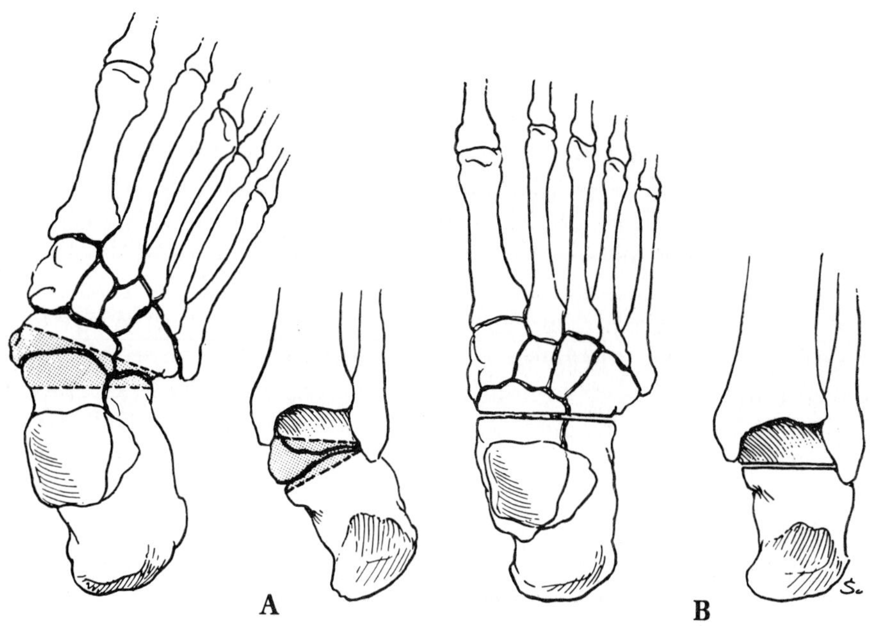

Figure 2. (Reproduced with permission from Crenshaw, A.H. (Ed.): *Campbell's Operative Orthopaedics*, Vol. 2, C.V. Mosby, St. Louis, 1971, p. 1527.)

1. Wedge-shaped section of bone is removed from the midtarsal region with the base on medial side of the foot (A).
2. Shaded area indicates the amount of bone removed.
3. Eversion of the os calcis is corrected by wedge-shaped resection of subtalar joint.
4. Position of bones after surgery (B).
5. Postoperative care same as triple arthrodesis without wedging.

II. Reconstruction for varus deformity

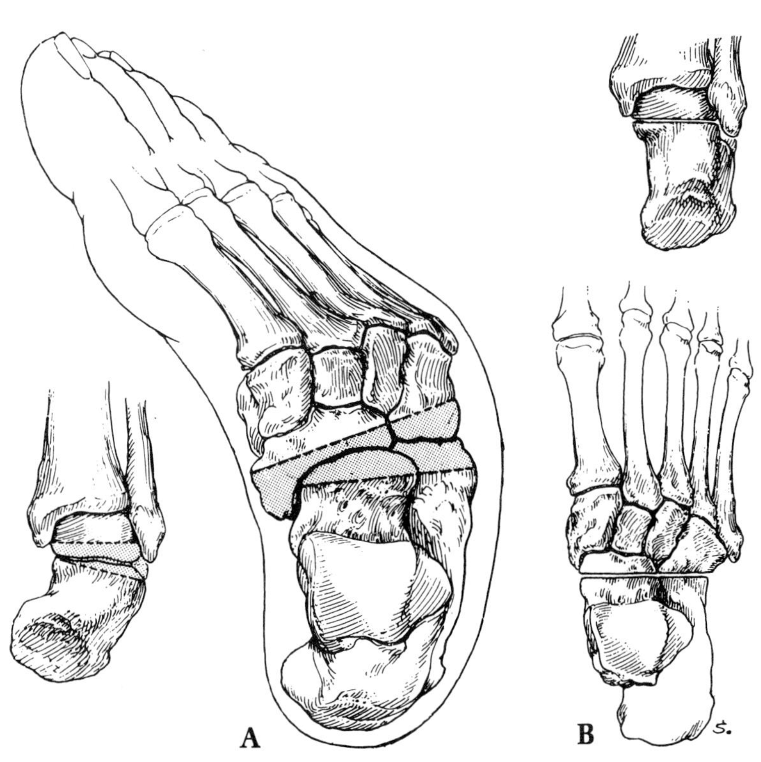

Figure 3. (Reproduced with permission from Crenshaw, A.H. (Ed.): *Campbell's Operative Orthopaedics*, Vol. 2, C.V. Mosby, St. Louis, 1971, p. 1527.)

1. Wedge-shaped section of bone is removed from the midtarsal region with the base on lateral side of the foot (A).
2. Shaded area indicates the amount of bone removed.
3. Inversion of the os calcis is corrected by wedge-shaped resection of subtalar joint.
4. Position of bones after surgery (B).
5. Postoperative care same as for triple arthrodesis without wedging.

Hoke's Triple Arthrodesis[4]

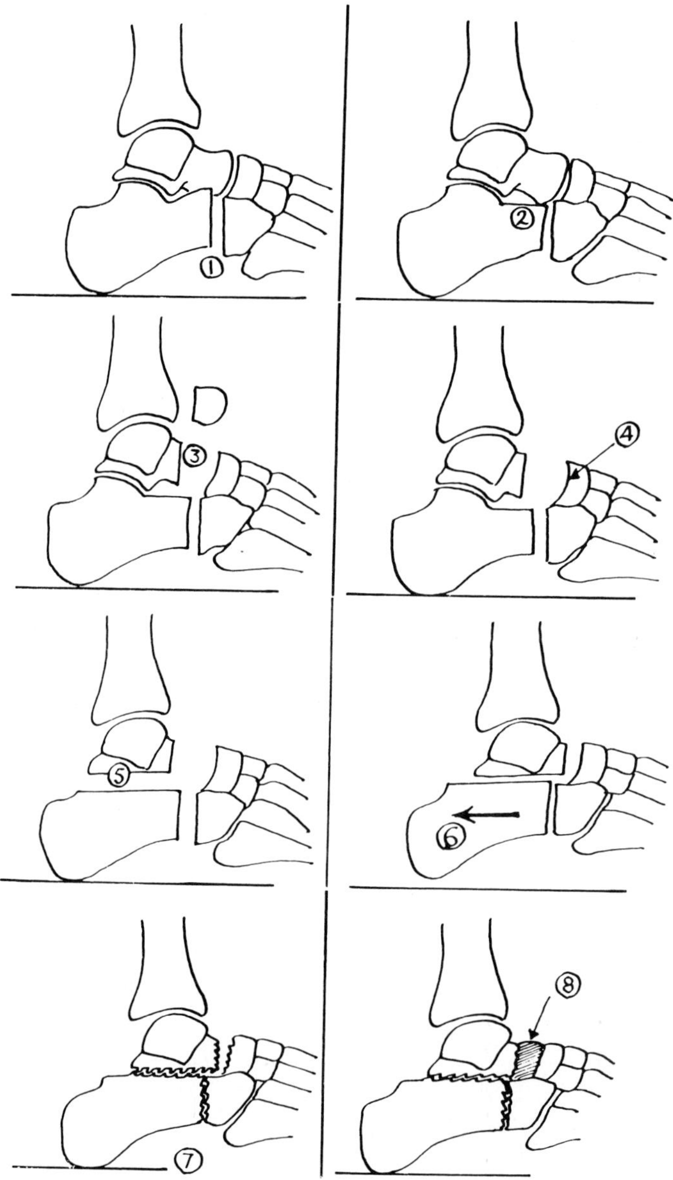

Figure 4. Technique of Hoke's triple arthrodesis. (1) First joint resected is the calcaneocuboid. (2) Second procedure is resection of promontory of os calcis. (3) Third procedure is resection of head and portion of neck of talus. (4) Fourth procedure is the resection of cartilage of navicular. (5) Fifth procedure is resection of cartilage of talus and os calcis (posterior subtalar joint). (6) Sixth procedure is adjustment of bones of foot on talus with posterior displacement to obtain tibiotalar balance. (7) Seventh procedure, "fish-scaling" of the resected joints. (8) Placement of talar head graft in predetermined position for correction of deformity. Following this all interspaces are loaded with fine small bone graft chips before soft tissue closure. (Reproduced with permission from Sideman, S.: Surgery of Poliomyelitis of the Lower Extremity, *Surg. Clin. N. Am.*, **45**:190, 1965.)

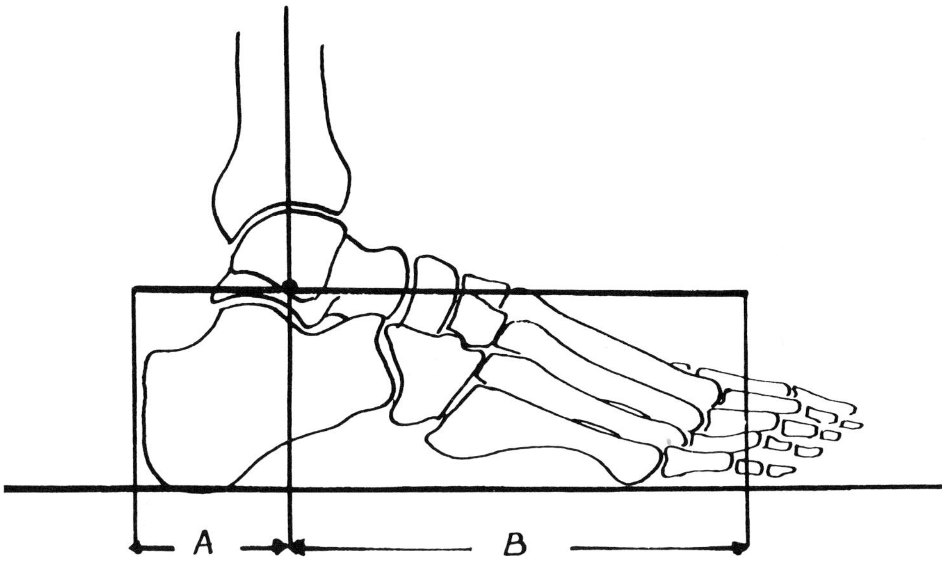

Figure 5a. Normal relations and tibiotalar balance. Note tibiotalar 90 degree angle. (Reproduced with permission from Sideman, S.: Surgery of Poliomyelitis of the Lower Extremity, *Surg. Clin. N. Am.*, **45**:193, 1965.)

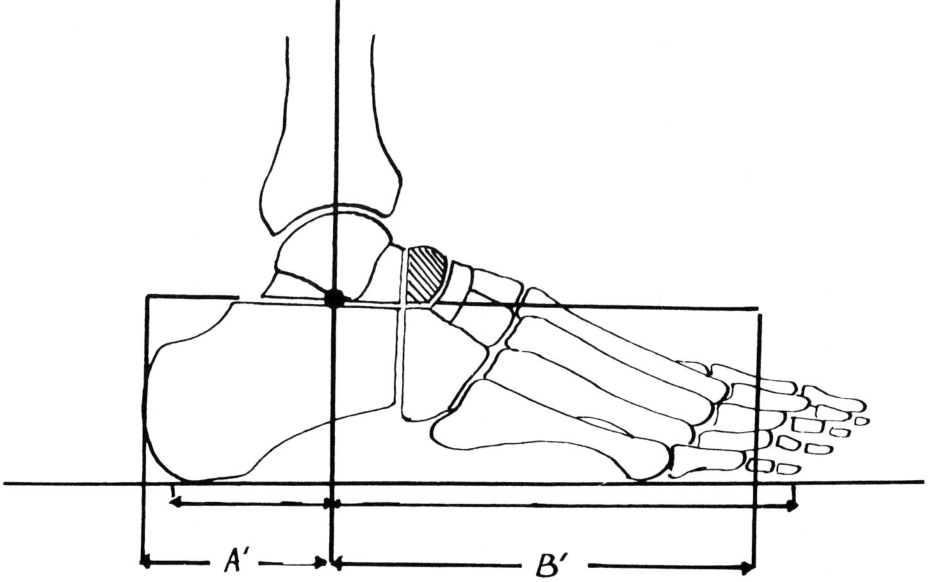

Figure 5b. Hoke triple corrected position with the shaded graft replacement after resection of the subtalar and calcaneocuboid joints. A′ and B′, replacement of foot on talus to balance ankle in neutral position for a nondeformed paralytic foot. Note tibiotalar 90 degree angle. (Reproduced with permission from Sideman, S.: Surgery of Poliomyelitis of the Lower Extremity, *Surg. Clin. N. Am.*, **45**:193, 1965.)

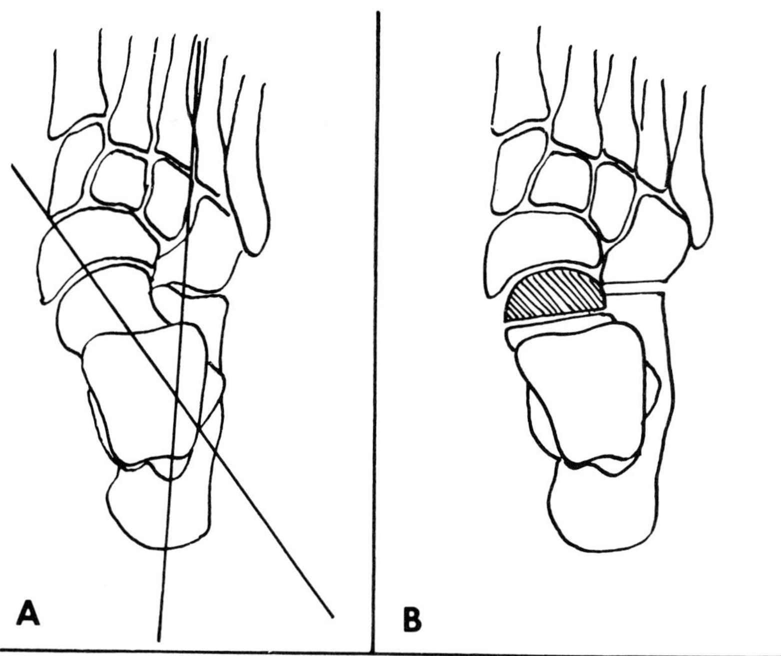

Figure 5c. (A) Normal angle of talonavicular calcaneus. (B) Placement of talar head graft after triple joint resection. No change in talonavicular calcaneus angle. (Reproduced with permission from Sideman, S.: Surgery of Poliomyelitis of the Lower Extremity, *Surg. Clin. N. Am.*, **45**:196, 1965.)

Technique

1. A 2½-inch oblique incision is made on the lateral aspect of the foot from the navicular bone at the point where the extensor tendons cross the talonavicular joint downward, across the middle of the sinus tarsi to the peroneal tendons 1 inch below the tip of the fibula. The tip of the fibula, the extensor digitorum tendon, the calcaneocuboid joint, and the peroneal tendons form a parallelogram, and this is bisected from the extensor tendon to the peroneal tendon across the sinus tarsi.
2. The skin incision is carried down through the subcutaneous fascia, and the soft, fatty, areolar tissue of the sinus tarsi is enucleated by passing the scalpel deep into the sinus tarsi and running it along the superior border of the os calcis and the inferior border of the talus. This mass of tissue is called the Hoke tonsil.
3. All soft tissue on the presenting surface of the os calcis and the neck and body of the talus are skeletonized carefully.
4. The cartilage of the approximating surfaces of the os calcis and cuboid are removed.

5. The promontory surface of the os calcis is completely removed across the superior surface of the bone at the point which brings the superior surface of the os calcis in a plane with the cuboid.
6. The neck of the talus is cut through, and the head and part of the neck of the talus are removed and placed in a basin of normal saline solution for later use. This exposes the articular surface of the navicular.
7. The cartilage is removed from the navicular with a curved gouge or osteotome.
8. The posterior subtalar joint is visualized by putting a periosteal elevator underneath the body of the talus and tilting it so that the surfaces of the subtalar joint are brought into view.
9. The cartilage from the talus and the superior surface of the os calcis is excised with an osteotome.
10. The lines of the osteotomy cuts are such that they are just deep enough to pick off the cartilage and enable a posterior displacement of the foot on the talus.
11. The presenting surfaces of the talus and the os calcis are fish-scaled with an osteotome, as are the contacting surface of the calcaneocuboid joint, the presenting surface of the navicular, the inferior surface of the body and part of the neck of the talus.
12. The head and neck of the talus are denuded of cartilage and cut to size for correct alignment of the foot on the talus.
13. Chips are taken from the head and neck of the talus, as well as fragments of bone scaled off the os calcis, talus, navicular, and cuboid, and placed in the space between the talus, os calcis, cuboid, and navicular.
14. A plaster of Paris cast is applied from the toes to above the knee. The cast is split, according to the technique of Hoke, and with a longitudinal saw the entire length of the cast is cut to the sheet wadding and lateral parallel cuts are made half-way through the cast. Cross cuts are made all the way through the cast in segments 2–2½ inches wide. These can be turned up and hinged on the lateral and medial saw cuts to allow for edema. These saw-cut segments can be turned down as the edema subsides and the cast maintained in its original contour.
15. After ten to fourteen days the cast is changed and the sutures are removed. A below-the-knee cast is applied. After four more weeks, a new cast is applied with a walking heel, and partial weight-bearing with crutches is started.
16. The complete cast is removed three to four months after surgery. This is followed by the use of an ace bandage until the edema subsides and the patient is able to bear weight without support (average four to six months postoperatively).

Hoke's Triple Arthrodesis for Calcaneus, Equinus, Varus, and Valgus Deformities

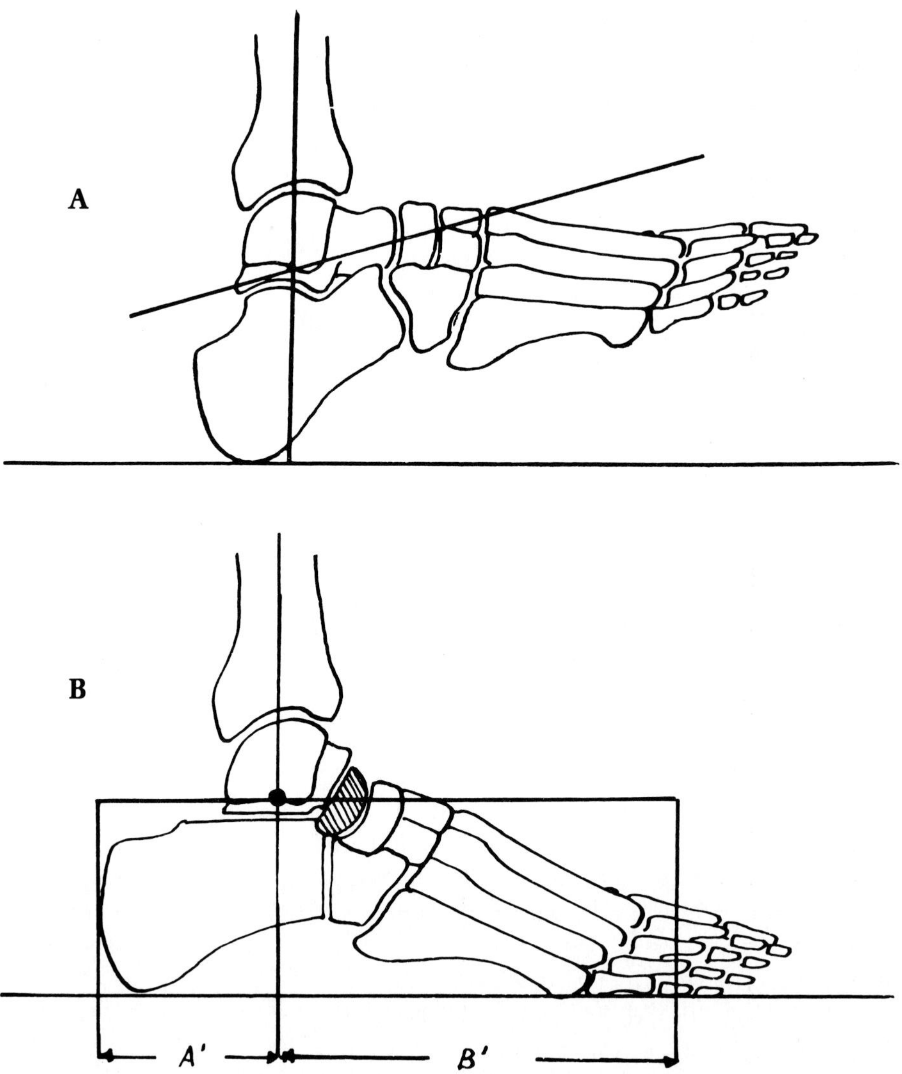

Figure 6. (A) Calcaneal foot. (B) Calcaneal foot corrected. (Reproduced with permission from Sideman, S.: Surgery of Poliomyelitis of the Lower Extremity, *Surg. Clin. N. Am.* **45**:195, 1965.)

1. *Calcaneus Deformity.* The forefoot is set on the talus with the talus in calcaneus, the foot at 90 degrees with the tibia, and the os calcis displaced posteriorly. In this way no further calcaneus deformity can develop because all the calcaneal dorsiflexion has been taken up in the talotibial joint.

The position is maintained when casting by pin fixation from the plantar surface through the heel, talus, and tibia.

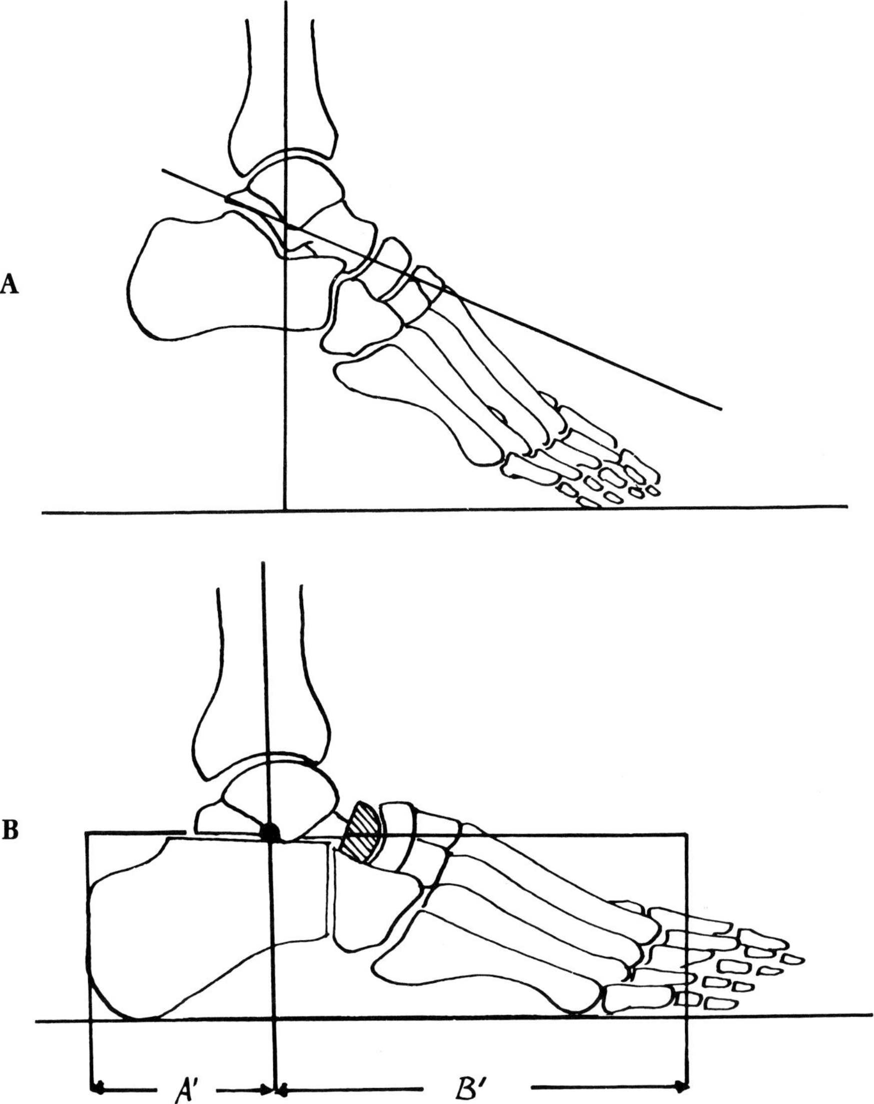

Figure 7. (A) Equinus foot. (B) Equinus foot corrected. (Reproduced with permission from Sideman, S.: Surgery of Poliomyelitis of the Lower Extremity, Surg. *Clin. N. Am.*, **45**:194, 1965.)

2. *Equinus Deformity.* The position of the navicular is such that the graft is placed inferior to the navicular and prevents the navicular from dropping into equinus.

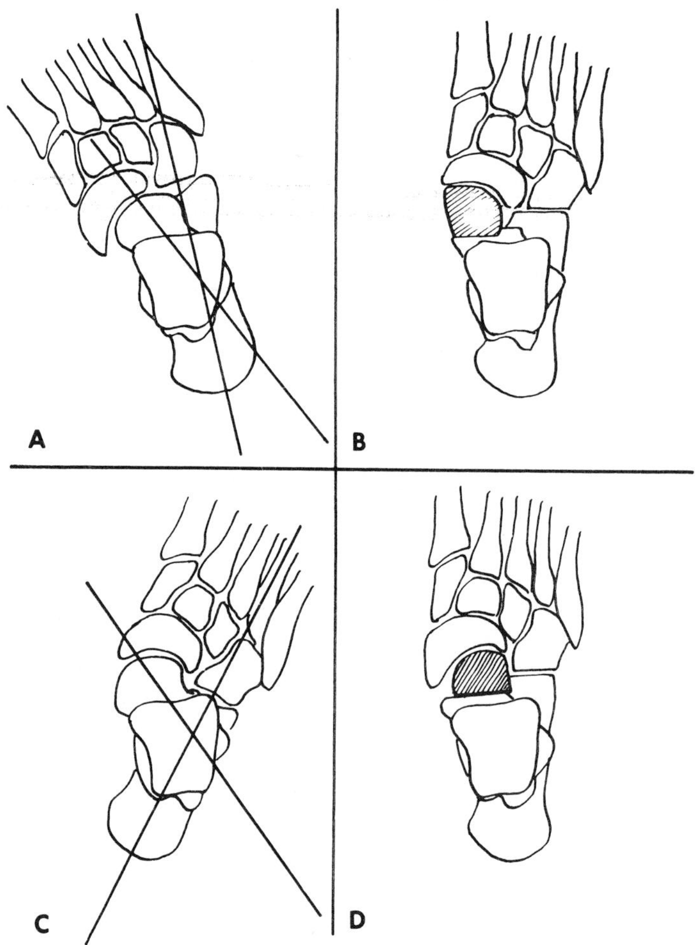

Figure 8. (A) Varus foot. (B) Varus foot corrected. (C) Valgus foot. (D) Valgus foot corrected. (Reproduced with permission from Sideman, S.: Surgery of Poliomyelitis of the Lower Extremity, *Surg. Clin. N. Am.*, **45**:197, 1965.)

3. *Varus Deformity.* The graft is placed in a position medially on the body of the talus, thereby preventing the foot from going into varus.
4. *Valgus Deformity.* The graft is placed laterally on the talus to prevent the forefoot from going into valgus.

References

1. Ryerson, E.W.: Arthrodesing operations on the feet. *J. Bone Jt. Surg.*, **41B**:524, 1923.
2. Goldstein, L.A., and Dickerson, R.C.: *Atlas of Orthopaedic Surgery*, Vol. 2, C.V. Mosby, St. Louis, 1974, pp. 894–897.
3. Crenshaw, A.H. (Ed.): *Campbell's Operative Orthopaedics*, Vol. 2, C.V. Mosby, St. Louis, 1971, p. 1523–1528.

4. Sideman, S.: Surgery of poliomyelitis of the lower extremity. *Surg. Clin. North Am.*, **45**:189–198, 1965.

Selected Bibliography

Hoke, M.: An operation for stabilizing the paralytic foot. *Am. J. Orthop. Surg.*, **41B**:524, 1923.

Larmon, W.A.: Arthrodesis of the joints of the lower extremity. *Surg. Clin. North Am.*, **45**:157–161, 1965.

Steindler, A.: *Orthopedic Operations*, Charles C Thomas, Springfield, Ill., 1940, pp. 328–330.

b. The head of the talus, the entire scaphoid bone, and the proximal cartilage coverings of the cuneiform bones are removed.
c. A cup-shaped depression is made at the ends of the cuneiform bones to fit them to the corresponding surface of the neck of the astragalus (talus).

5. The ligaments between the talus and the os calcis are divided, the two bones are pried apart by means of a gouge, and the adjoining surfaces of the talus and os calcis are resected as in the subtalar arthrodesis.
6. It is now possible to displace the foot backward so that the neck of the talus rests upon the cuneiform bones while the bodies of the cuboid and os calcis also come into apposition.
7. The extensor brevis digitorum is now replaced and the wound is closed.
8. The arch of the foot is now much more symmetrical, with the weight-bearing center at the summit of the arch.
9. Casting and postoperative care are the same as for triple arthrodesis (Chapter 6).

Putti Procedure[3,4]

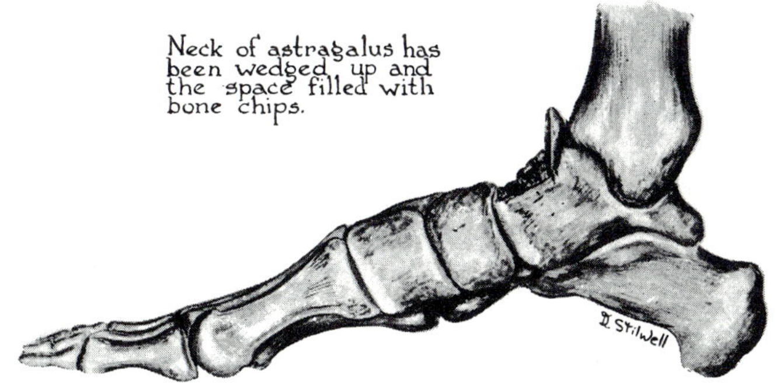

Figure 2. Anterior bone block of ankle. (Reproduced with permission from Steindler, A.: *Orthopedic Operations: Indications, Technique, and End Results,* Charles C Thomas, Springfield, Ill., 1940, p. 342.)

1. A longitudinal incision is made in front of the ankle joint.
2. The extensors are defined and retracted until the lower end of the tibia, as well as the anterior surface of the body of the talus, are exposed.
3. A transverse cut is made with a chisel at about the middle of the body of the talus.
4. The trough produced is filled with bone chips, and a wall is piled up against the anterior edge of the tibia.
5. Soft parts are sutured over the bone to keep the implant in place. Skin closure effected in the usual manner.
6. The foot is casted at right angles, and walking is permitted in the cast after four weeks.

Whitman Talectomy (Astragalectomy)[5,6,7]

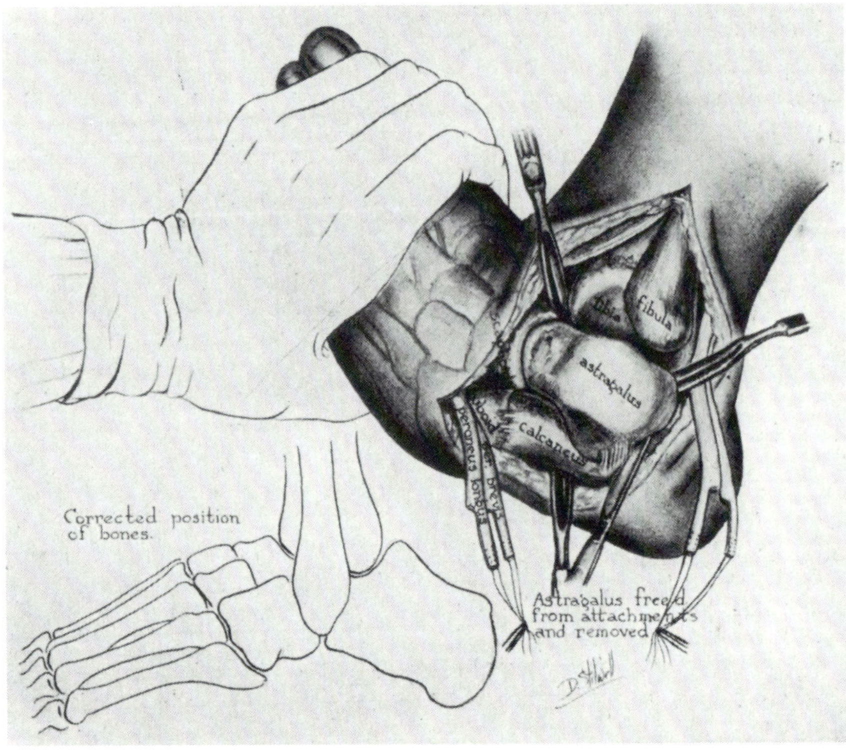

Figure 3. (Reproduced with permission from Steindler, A.: *Orthopedic Operations: Indications, Technique, and End Results,* Charles C Thomas, Springfield, Ill., 1940, p. 343.)

1. The line of incision begins at a point 1 inch above the external malleolus and runs downward behind the fibula and forward ¾ inch below the malleolus and then in a curve over the dorsum of the foot to the head of the talus (Kocher's incision).
2. The sheaths of the peronei are opened, and the tendons are secured by forceps divided below the malleolus and reflected.
3. The external ligament and the interossei ligament are then divided.
4. Proceeding underneath the extensor tendons, dissect the talus starting from the body and proceeding to the neck and head. The foot is then given a forceful inward twist and the whole joint is widely opened so that the head and neck of the talus may be freed all around until the entire bone is freed from its ligamentous attachments and removed.
5. A new articulation for the mortise of the tibia and fibula to articulate with the floor is prepared as follows:
   a. A thin section of bone is cut from the adjoining outer surfaces of the cuboid and the talus, and the soft tissues are stripped off the internal aspect of the scaphoid.
   b. The internal malleolus is carefully dissected out, and the surrounding soft tissue is also stripped back.

c. The articular surfaces are removed from both the internal and external malleoli, and they are shaped to fit into the new places of the articulation when the foot is displaced backward.

6. The foot is now placed in its new relation to the leg by displacing the foot 1–1½ inches. The mortise of the malleoli now becomes adapted to the junction of the calcaneus and the cuboid on the outside, and to a point directly behind the inner border of the scaphoid on the inside of the foot. The anterior surface of the tibia now lies directly behind the level of Chopart's joint, and the heel protrudes backward. The malleoli rest deeply and firmly in their new positions. *This is the most important part of the operation because upon it depends the static rearrangement of the foot.*
7. The peroneal tendons are reunited or inserted into the tendo Achillis, and the wound is closed.
8. A plaster of Paris cast is applied from the toes to above the slightly flexed knee, with the foot in plantar flexion and a very slight valgus position. The limb is then held in a hammock and counterbalanced.
9. The total period of fixation is from two to three months. During that time the cast is changed to reduce the amount of plantar flexion. After removal of the cast, the patient is able to wear an ordinary boot.

References

1. Dunn, N.: *On Stabilizing Operations in the Treatment of Paralytic Deformities of the Feet,* Bristol, England, 1922.
2. Dunn, N.: Calcaneo-cavus and its treatment. *Am. J. Orthoped. Surg.,* December, 1919.
3. Putti, V., and Mezzari, A.: L'arthrodesi tibio-astragalea secondo Putti. *Chir. Org. Mov.,* **8**:5, 1924.
4. Crenshaw, A.H. (Ed.): *Campbell's Operative Orthopaedics,* Vol. 2, C.V. Mosby, St. Louis, 1971, pp. 1528–1529, 1572–1574.
5. Whitman, R.: Further observations on the operative treatment of paralytic talipes calcaneus. *Am. J. Orthop. Surg.,* **8**:137, 1910.
6. Whitman, R.: Astragalectomy and backward displacement of the foot. *J. Bone Jt. Surg.* **20**:266, .922.
7. Steindler, A.: *Orthopedic Operations: Indications, Technique, and End Results,* Charles C Thomas, Springfield, Ill., 1940, pp. 333, 342–344.

CHAPTER 8

Talipes Equinus Deformity

Osseous talipes equinus is a deformity involving both the foot and the ankle, in which the foot deformity is characterized by a plantar flexion. This deformity does not permit the foot to dorsiflex at least 10 degrees at the ankle joint with the knee extended or flexed when the subtalar joint is in a neutral position. Biomechanical evaluation, gait analysis and roentgenology will enable the surgeon to make a diagnosis of gastrocnemius equinus, gastro-soleus equinus or osseous equinus.

Congenital gastrocnemius and gastro-soleus equinus can be corrected by soft tissue procedures as discussed in Chapters 3 and 4. Poor results from soft tissue procedures are attributable to osseous equinus that was not diagnosed prior to surgery. The arthrodeses discussed in this chapter are for the correction of osseous talipes equinus. In this deformity there is a limitation of dorsiflexion due to structural bony deformity, usually of the talar dome, which may cause a disabling degenerative arthritis at the ankle joint.

In addition to the procedures detailed in Chapters 6 and 7, there are several techniques that have been developed in combination with triple arthrodesis to correct the talipes equinus deformity.

With the Lambrinudi procedure, as with the Naughton Dunn technique discussed in Chapter 7, it is essential to make a preoperative blueprint from a tracing of a lateral x-ray film of the deformed foot. The x-ray should be taken with the foot in extreme plantar flexion. The tracing thus obtained is cut into three sections at the edges of the demarcation of the subtalar and midtarsal joints. The line on the tracing that shows the articulation of the talus is kept, but those that represent the distal and plantar aspects of the talus are cut so that the navicular and calcaneocuboid joints can be fitted to the foot in slight equinus. In relation to the leg, this angle should be between 5 and 10 degrees, unless the foot has become shortened, in which case a more extreme angle of equinus may be necessary. These aspects of the operative procedure can be planned with great accuracy from the paper tracing obtained before operation.

The posterior Campbell bone block, an osteoplastic procedure, was developed to check plantar flexion of the foot. This is accomplished surgically by forming an extra-articular bone block, by which the foot is stabilized against lateral and medial movement. This technique is generally employed in combination with arthrodesis, but dorsiflexion of the ankle joint is maintained.

Lambrinudi Procedure[1]

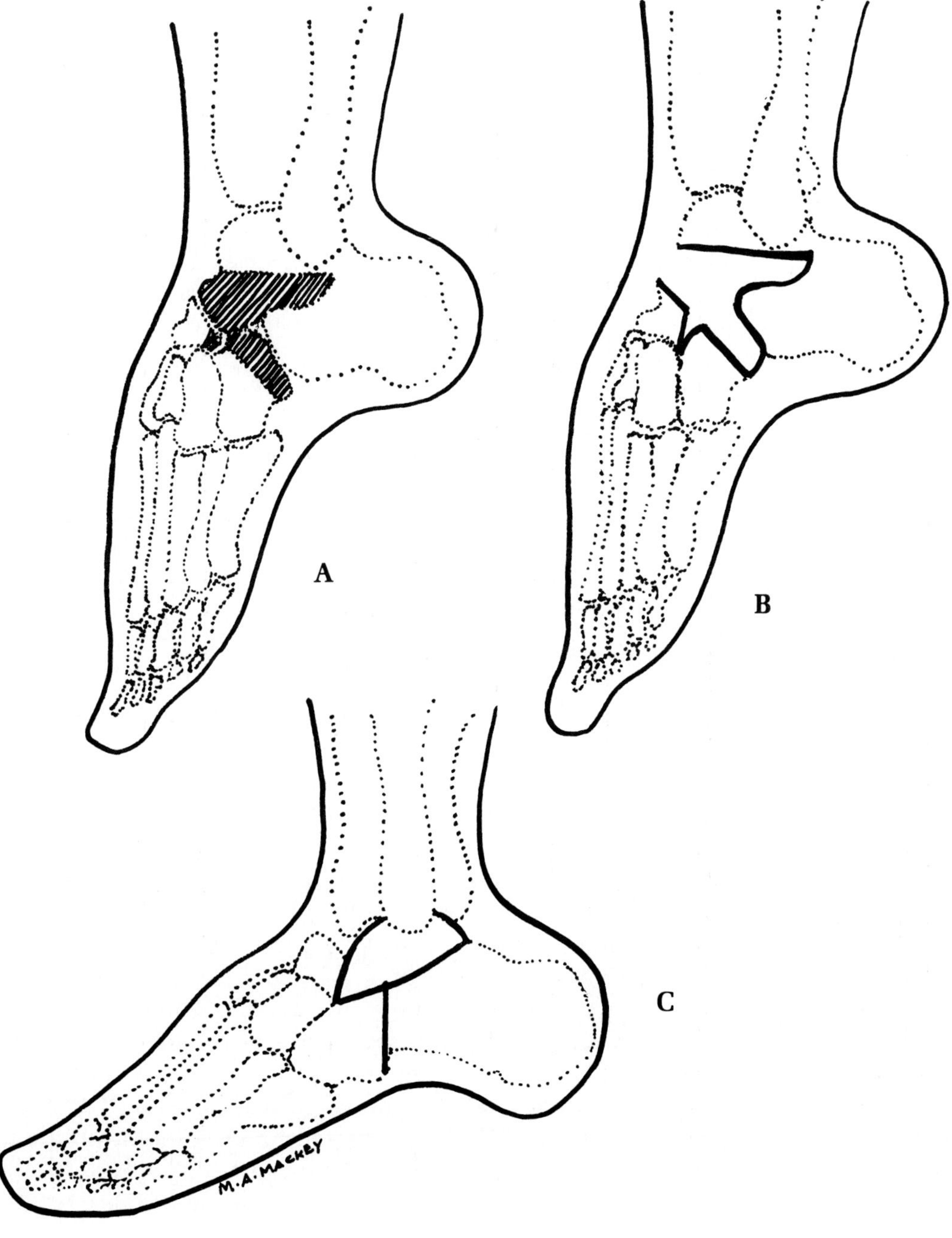

Figure 1. Lambrinudi operation for talipes equinus. (A) Shaded area indicates portion of bone and cartilage to be resected. (B) Portion of bone and cartilage resected. (C) Equinus and calcaneus deformities corrected by wedging the sharp distal margin of the remaining portion of the talus into the prepared trough in the navicular and opposing the raw osseous surfaces of the talus, calcaneus and cuboid.

1. The tarsus is exposed through a long, lateral curved incision.
2. The peroneal tendons are sectioned by a Z-shaped cut.
3. The talonavicular and calcaneocuboid joints are opened, and the interosseous and fibular collateral ligaments are divided to permit complete medial dislocation of the tarsus at the subtalar joint.
4. The predetermined wedge of bone is removed from the plantar and distal parts of the neck and body of the talus with a small handsaw.
5. The cartilage and bone are removed from the superior surface of the calcaneus to form a plane parallel with the longitudinal axis of the foot.
6. A V-shaped trough is made transversely in the inferior part of the proximal navicular, and the calcaneocuboid joint is denuded of enough bone to correct any lateral deformity.
7. Firmly wedge the sharp distal margin of the remaining part of the talus into the prepared trough in the navicular and appose the calcaneus and talus, taking care to place the distal margin of the talus well medially in the trough, otherwise the position of the foot will not be satisfactory. No attempt should be made to compensate in the foot for any tibial torsion.
8. The talus is now locked in the ankle joint in complete equinus, and the foot cannot be plantar flexed.
9. The peroneal tendons are sutured.
10. Wound closed in the routine manner.
11. After treatment and casting are the same as for triple arthrodesis.

Posterior Campbell Bone Block[2]

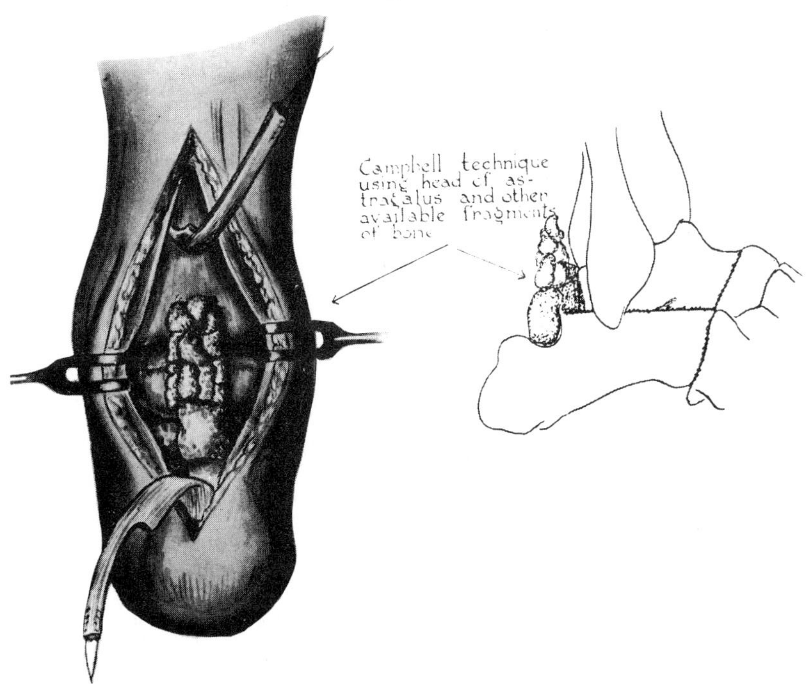

Figure 2a. Posterior bone block of ankle. Showing use of head of astragalus and other available fragments of bone. (Reproduced with permission from Steindler, A.: *Orthopedic Operations: Indications, Technique, and End Results*, Charles C Thomas, Springfield, Ill., 1940, p. 340.)

1. An incision 3–4 inches long is made along the medial border of the tendo Achillis from its insertion in the calcaneus proximally in a straight line.
2. If the tendo Achillis is contracted, it is lengthened by Z-plasty; otherwise, it is retracted laterally.
3. A straight incision is made through the deep structures in the midline to the posterior surface of the ankle joint.
4. The tendon of the flexor longus hallucis is retracted medially.
5. Using a periosteal elevator, a pyramidal space is cleared, and the posterior surfaces of the tibia, ankle joint, and subtalar joint and the superior surface of the calcaneus are exposed.
6. The foot is dorsiflexed to bring the posterior surface of the talus into view.
7. The posterior surface of the talus is resected, and immediately below it a wedge is excavated from the superior surface of the calcaneus so that the posterior surface of the remaining part of the talus makes a smooth coronal plane with one side of the cavity in the calcaneus. *Care should be taken to avoid denuding the posterior surface of the tibia; otherwise, the bone block may unite with it and fuse the ankle joint.*
8. A triple arthrodesis is usually performed, and the fragments of bone removed may be used for the bone block. The largest piece is inserted into the cavity, and small particles of bone are arranged in a pyramid above the wedge (head of talus).
9. If the tendo Achillis has been lengthened by Z-plasty, it is sutured in the corrected position.
10. Wound closed in the routine manner.
11. After care and casting are the same as for a triple arthrodesis. The foot is casted at an exact right angle to the leg; otherwise, a calcaneus deformity will occur.
12. *Modifications.* When the foot has already been stabilized, several flaps of bone are reflected anteriorly and superiorly from the superior surface of the calcaneus. *Steindler modification.* A tibial bone graft (instead of bone chips) is implanted into a groove made in the calcaneus immediately behind the posterior border of the talus.

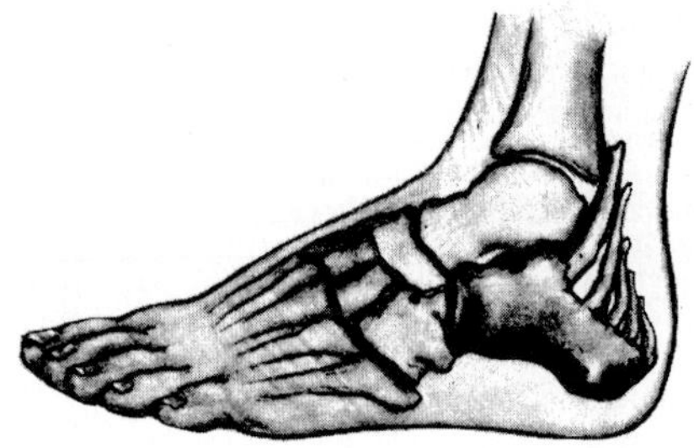

Figure 2b. Posterior bone block for talipes equinus. Bone block operation has been carried out by reflecting bone superiorly and anteriorly from superior surface of calcaneus. (Reproduced with permission from Crenshaw, A.H. (Ed.): *Campbell's Operative Orthopaedics,* Vol. 2, C.V. Mosby, St. Louis, 1971, p. 1551.)

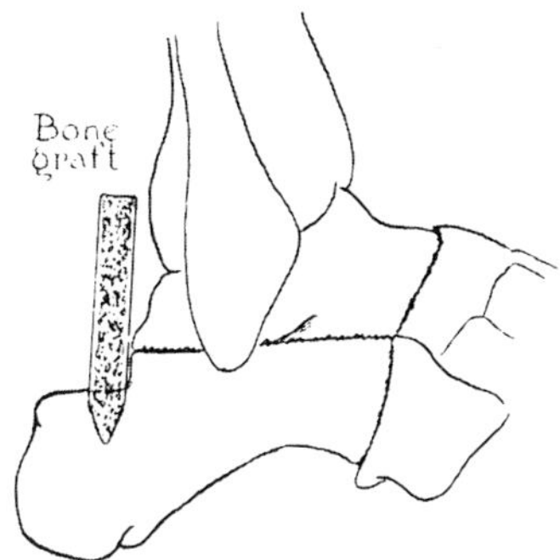

Figure 2c. Posterior bone block of ankle showing use of a tibial graft. (Reproduced with permission from Steindler, A.: *Orthopedic Operations: Indications, Technique, and End Results*, Charles C Thomas, Springfield, Ill., 1940, p. 340.)

Gill Procedure[3]

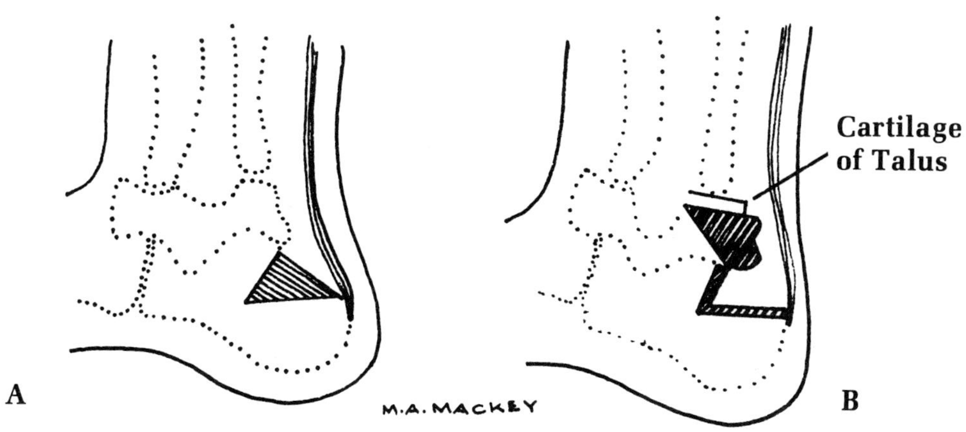

Figure 3. Posterior bone block for talipes equinus by Gill technique. (A) Shaded portion is bone wedge to be resected from the calcaneus just anterior to the attachment of the tendo Achillis. (B) Wedge of bone taken from calcaneus is placed into wedge-shaped space formed when a thin layer of bone is lifted from the posterior lip of the talus.

1. A longitudinal incision approximately 3–4 inches long is made along the medial border of the tendo Achillis from its insertion in the calcaneus proximally.
2. The tendo Achillis is divided by a Z-shaped cut.
3. The ankle and superior aspect of the calcaneus are exposed.
4. The foot is dorsiflexed as much as possible to bring into view the posterior part of the superior articular surface of the talus.

5. With a broad, thin osteotome (Swedish osteotome) the cartilage with a thin layer of bone is lifted from the posterior of the talus and apposed to the posterior lip of the talus to form the apex of a wedge-shaped space beneath the cartilage anterior to the posterior lip of the tibia.
6. A wedge of bone is excised from the superior aspect of the calcaneus and inserted into the space, while the foot is held in dorsiflexion.
7. The tendo Achillis and the incision are sutured in the usual manner.
8. The foot is immobilized in a plaster cast for three months.

References

1. Lambrinudi, C.: New operation on drop foot. *Br. J. Surg.*, **15**:193–200, 1927.
2. Campbell, W.C.: Operation for the correction of drop foot. *J. Bone Jt. Surg.*, **21**:4, 1923.
3. Gill, A.B.: An operation to make a posterior bone block at the ankle to limit foot drop. *J. Bone Jt. Surg.*, **15**:166–170, 1933.

Selected Bibliography

Crenshaw, A.H. (Ed.): *Campbell's Operative Orthopaedics,* Vol. 2, C.V. Mosby, St. Louis, 1971, pp. 1550–1554.

DuVries, H.L.: *Surgery of the Foot,* 2 ed., C.V. Mosby, St. Louis, 1965, pp. 504–508.

Hart, V.L.: Lambrinudi operation for drop foot. *J. Bone Jt. Surg.* **22**:937–941, 1940.

Melillo, T.V.: Gastrocnemius equinus — Its diagnosis and treatment. *Arch. Pod. Med. and Foot Surg.,* **2**:159–205, 1975.

McGlamry, E.D.: *Reconstructive Surgery of the Foot and Leg,* Intercontinental Medical Book Corporation, New York, 1974, pp. 275-282.

Steindler, A.: *Orthopedic Operations: Indications, Technique, and End Results,* Charles C Thomas, Springfield, Ill., 1940, pp. 340–341.

Suppan, R.J.: Bone block procedures for drop foot. *J. Foot Surg.,* **16**:132–135, 1977.

CHAPTER 9

Calcaneocavus Deformity

Talipes calcaneocavus is a paralytic deformity caused by paralysis of the triceps surae. The tendo Achillis is thin and elongated since the long dorsiflexors of the foot at the ankle remain functional and unapposed. Because of the paralysis, the calcaneus cannot be stabilized nor can the body weight be borne on the metatarsal heads. The push-off in walking is lost, causing the calcaneus to rotate as its posterior end is pulled plantarly by the long and short toe flexors, the lumbricales and the interossei causing the development of a cavus deformity. With the development of a forefoot equinus and unapposed rotation of the calcaneus, the plantar fascia becomes contracted and, with growth, structural changes occur in the bones and joints.

Paralytic calcaneocavus defects have a shortening effect on the heel, and to compensate for this defect it is necessary to displace the foot posteriorly so that the lengthened calcaneus can function as a true lever. With this redistribution of weight, less muscle power is necessary for push-off during walking.

Tendon transfers are indicated in the skeletally immature foot to keep the deformity from increasing or to correct a severe deformity to prevent damaging the bones. After skeletal maturity, foot stabilization procedures as discussed in this chapter will be necessary.

With triple arthrodesis, posterior displacement is effected at the subtalar joint. However, if the disability is severe and muscles involved in tendon transfer are weak, a pantalar arthrodesis is required. Miller,[1] Irwin,[2] and Goldner[3] recommend manipulative therapy after the stabilization procedure has been performed.

A modified triple arthrodesis, the "beak" procedure, was developed by Siffert, Forster, and Nachamie[4] to improve the conformation of the foot with calcaneocavus deformity. By this technique talar reconstruction is accomplished in such a way that the soft tissues on the superior talar surface are preserved to maintain circulation to the talar head. Resection of the inferior talar head involves the construction of a beak-like projection below the talar head, anterior to the ankle.

A third procedure, developed by Jones, is a two-stage surgical technique.[5] Stage 1 involves correction of the cavus deformity by removal of a single wedge of bone at the apex of the cavus defect. This procedure accentuates the calcaneus deformity. Four weeks after the first procedure, the second operation is performed to correct the calcaneal deformity by arthrodesis of the ankle joint.

Triple Arthrodesis for Calcaneocavus Deformity[6]

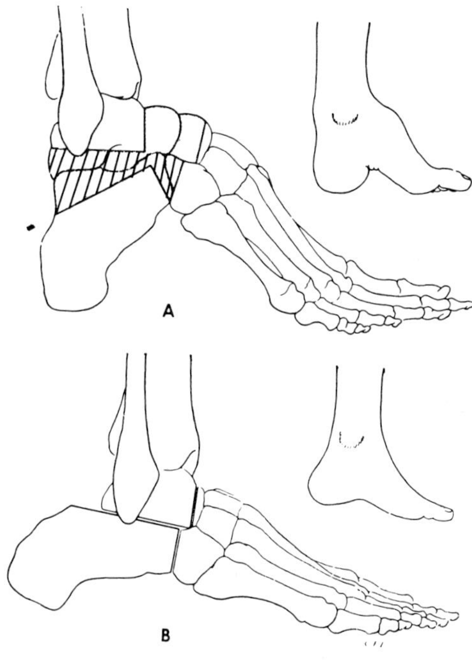

Figure 1. (A) *Shaded area,* amount of bone resected. (B) Position of bones after surgery; note that foot has been displaced posteriorly at subtalar joint. (Reproduced with permission from Crenshaw, A.H. (Ed.): *Campbell's Operative Orthopaedics,* Vol. 2, C.V. Mosby, St. Louis, 1971, p. 1570.)

1. Steindler stripping (Chapter 11) is performed to release the contracted soft tissue bridging the longitudinal arch. The cavus deformity is then forcibly corrected as much as possible.
2. The calcaneocuboid, talonavicular, and subtalar joints are exposed through the same incision used for triple arthrodesis (Chapter 6).
3. With an osteotome, remove from the talonavicular and calcaneocuboid joints a wedge-shaped section of bone with its base anterior and large enough to correct any residual cavus deformity.
4. The forefoot is then dorsiflexed and the raw surfaces apposed to determine whether the cavus deformity is corrected.
5. If not, the subtalar joint is exposed, and a wedge of bone is removed with its base posterior to correct the deformity.
6. Be sure that all bone surfaces fit together well and that the foot is in satisfactory position.
7. Closure is effected in the usual manner.
8. A cast is applied with the foot in moderate equinus and the knee in slight

flexion. Firm pressure is exerted on the sole of the foot while the plaster is setting to stretch the plantar structures as much as possible.

9. At ten to fourteen days, the cast is removed, the foot inspected, and x-ray films are taken. If the position is not satisfactory, the foot should be manipulated with the patient under general anaesthesia. A new cast, snug but properly padded, is then applied and molded to the contour of the foot.
10. After care is the same as for triple arthrodesis.

Siffert, Forster, and Nachamie Procedure[4,7]

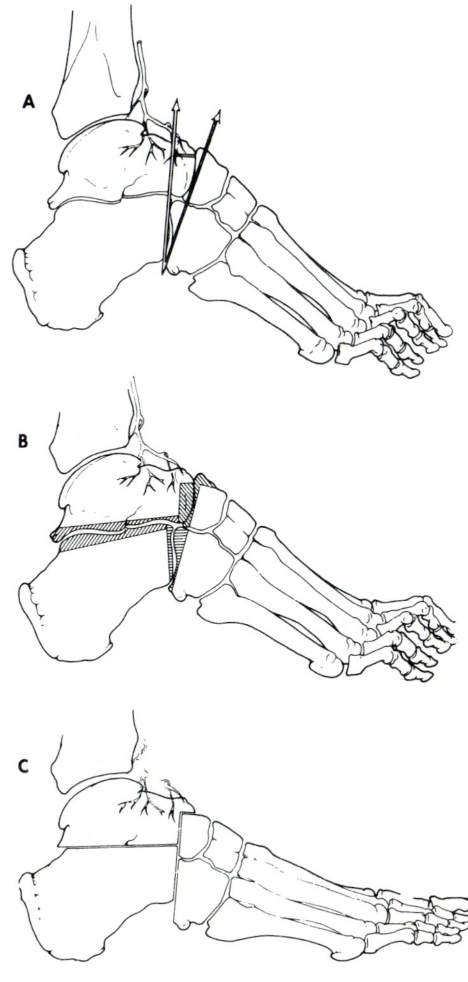

Figure 2. Triple arthrodesis for severe cavus deformity. (A) *Arrows,* wedge of bone to be removed by osteotomy. Notice that superior part of talar head is retained to form "beak". (B) *Shaded areas,* bone to be resected from region of midtarsal and subtalar joints. Notice that dorsal cortex of navicular is included. (C) Final position of foot; forefoot has been displaced plantarward and navicular has been locked beneath remaining part of talar head. (Courtesy of Dr. Robert S. Siffert and Dr. Jacob F. Katz. Reproduced with permission from DePalma, A.F. (Ed.): *Clinical Orthopaedics and Related Research,* Vol. 45, J.B. Lippincott, Philadelphia, 1966.)

1. Through the incision used for ordinary triple arthrodesis (Chapter 6), the calcaneocuboid, talonavicular, and subtalar joints are exposed.
2. The cartilage of the calcaneocuboid and subtalar joints is removed.
3. The dorsal cortex of the navicular is excised.
4. A wedge of bone is removed by osteotomy of the anterior aspect of the calcaneus, the posterior aspect of the navicular, and the inferior aspect of the talar head and neck. The osteotomy is started inferiorly and carried superiorly to the inferior surface of the talus. The inferior part of the talar head and neck is resected to form a beak, leaving undisturbed the soft tissue structures on the superior surface of the talus anterior to the ankle joint.
5. The forefoot is displaced plantarward to lock the navicular beneath the remaining part of the talar head and neck.
6. With the bones fitting together snugly, the position is maintained manually by applying slight pressure beneath the forefoot while the cast is being applied. If the fit is not snug, fix the talus to the navicular by a staple if desired, and if necessary fix the talus to the calcaneus.
7. After care is the same as for triple arthrodesis.

Jones Procedure for Calcaneocavus[5,8]

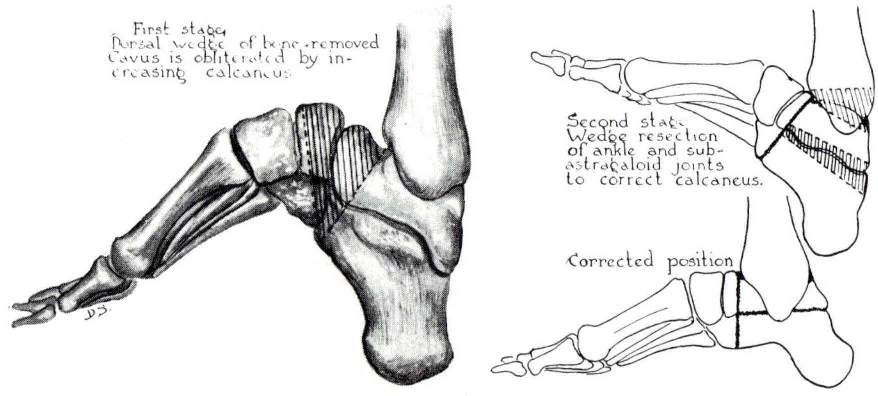

Fig. 151.—Jones' operation for calcaneo-cavus.

Figure 3. (Reproduced with permission from Steindler, A.: *Orthopedic Operations: Indications, Technique, and End Results,* Charles C Thomas, Springfield, Ill., 1940, p. 334.)

Stage 1

1. A Steindler stripping (see Chapter 2) is performed to release the contracted soft tissue bridging the longitudinal arch. The cavus deformity is then forcibly corrected as much as possible.
2. A three-inch incision is made on the inner border of the foot, and the soft parts are separated from the tarsus above and below from the inner to the outer side.
3. A V-shaped portion of bone is removed dorsally, corresponding to the apex of the cavus deformity.

4. Then, by strongly dorsiflexing the foot, it is possible to obliterate the cavus, thereby increasing the calcaneus deformity.
5. Closure is effected in the usual manner, and a cast is applied with the foot in calcaneus and the knee in slight flexion.

Stage 2 (Performed four weeks later)

1. A longitudinal incision is made in the center of the back of the heel opposite the ankle joint.
2. The tendo Achillis is retracted medially.
3. The ankle joint is opened and a wedge is taken from the tibia and the talus, with its base posteriorly.
4. The articular surfaces of the tibia and fibula are denuded.
5. The foot is brought into a right angle to the leg, thereby closing the wedge and correcting the calcaneus deformity.
6. Closure is effected in the usual manner, and a cast is applied with the foot at a right angle to the leg and the knee slightly flexed.
7. After care is the same as for triple arthrodesis.

References

1. Miller, O.L.: Surgical management of pes calcaneus, *J. Bone Jt. Surg.*, **18**:169, 1936.
2. Irwin, C.E.: The calcaneus foot. A revision. *American Academy of Orthopaedic Surgeons Instructional Course Lectures*, Vol. 15, J.W. Edwards, Ann Arbor, Mich., 1958.
3. Goldner, J.L., and Irwin, C.E.: Paralytic deformities of the foot. *American Academy of Orthopaedic Surgeons Instructional Course Lectures*, Vol. 5, J.W. Edwards, Ann Arbor, Mich., 1948.
4. Siffert, R.S., Forster, R.I., and Nachamie, B.: "Beak" triple arthrodesis for correction of severe cavus deformity. In A.F. De Palma (Ed.): *Clinical Orthopaedics and Related Research*, Vol. 45, J.P. Lippincott, Philadelphia, 1966.
5. Jones, R., and Lovett, R.W.: *Orthopaedic Surgery*, 2 ed., Wm. Wood, Baltimore, 1933.
6. Crenshaw, A.H. (Ed.): *Campbell's Operative Orthopaedics*, Vol. 2, C.V. Mosby, St. Louis, 1971, pp. 1569–1571.
7. De Palma, A.F. (Ed.): *Clinical Orthopaedics and Related Research*, Vol. 45, J.B. Lippincott, Philadelphia, 1966.
8. Steindler, A.: *Orthopedic Operations: Indications, Technique, and End Results*, Charles C Thomas, Springfield, Ill., 1940, p. 334.

CHAPTER 10

Equinovalgus Deformity

Correction of an equinovalgus deformity is most satisfactorily accomplished by triple arthrodesis with specific modifications to fit individual cases. To correct the valgus of the heel and to eliminate or reduce pronation and abduction of the subtalar joint it is necessary to remove a wedge of bone from the medial aspect of the talonavicular joint. Elongation of the lateral edge of the foot is then accomplished by packing bone chips around the calcaneocuboid joint. By thus elongating the foot, the forefoot becomes abducted and supinated, which brings the heel into both varus and valgus, and the heads of the first and fifth metatarsals lie in the same plane.

To accomplish this complex type of correction, Grice and Green devised a two-stage procedure that involves extra-articular fusion of the subtalar joint, followed six to eight weeks later by transfer of the peroneus longus and brevis tendons. In some cases the stage 2 operation will be deferred if equinus must be corrected by wedge casting or if the foot must be mobilized so that muscles can be strengthened. In other cases, when the patient is too young to participate intelligently in postoperative therapy for retraining muscle groups, the operation should be postponed until the child develops this ability.

Grice and Green Extra-articular Subtalar Arthrodesis[1-5]

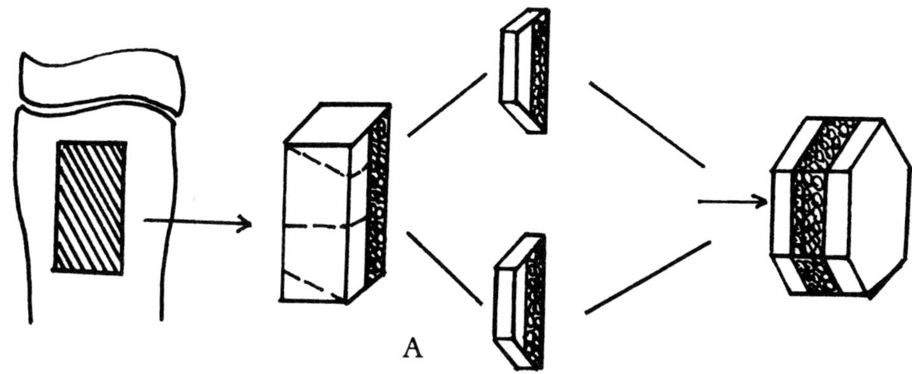

Figure 1. Grice and Green extra-articular subtalar arthrodesis. (A) Full thickness tibial graft shaped for insertion. *(Continued on next page.)*

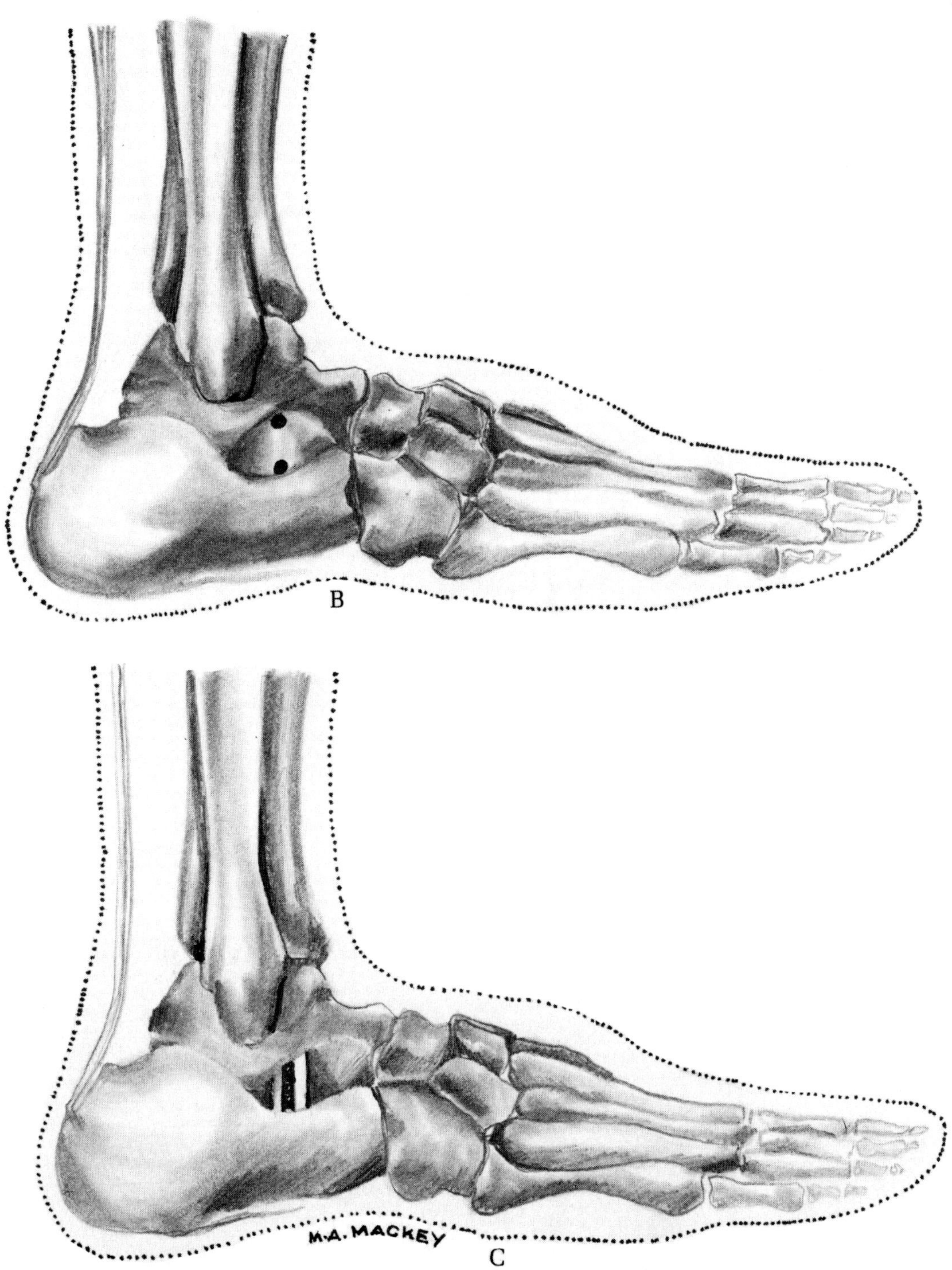

Figure 1 (continued). Grice and Green extra-articular subtalar arthrodesis. (B) Proper location of slots in the roof and floor of the sinus tarsi. (C) Tibial graft has been placed so that its vertical axis is parallel to the long axis of the tibia when the foot and ankle are in its neutral position.

1. A short, curved lateral incision is made directly over the subtalar joint.
2. The interosseous talocalcaneal ligament overlying the joint is exposed and cut in the direction of its fibers.
3. The fatty and ligamentous tissue is dissected from the sinus tarsi.
4. The extensor brevis digitorum is incised at its origin and reflected distally.
5. The foot is placed in equinus and inversion so that the calcaneus can be rotated into its normal position beneath the talus. If the deformity is severe and of long duration it may be necessary to divide the posterior capsule of the subtalar or remove a small amount of bone laterally from beneath the anterosuperior articular surface of the calcaneus before normal alignment can be restored.
6. A broad periosteal elevator is inserted into the sinus tarsi to block the subtalar joint to determine the size and optimum position of the grafts, as well as to demonstrate the stability they will afford.
7. If the distal end of the calcaneus cannot be held beneath the talus despite correction of the valgus deformity, a screw is inserted through a small anterior incision to transfix the anterior talocalcaneal articulation.
8. A thin layer of cortical bone is removed from the inferior surface of the talus and the superior surface of the calcaneus to prepare beds for the grafts.
9. From the anteriomedial surface of the proximal tibial metaphysis a block of bone (3.5–4.5 cm long and 1.5 cm wide) is removed to provide two grafts.
10. The grafts are cut like trapezoids to fit the prepared bed. The corners of the broad base of each graft are rongeured so that each can be countersunk into cancellous bone, thereby preventing their lateral displacement after surgery.
11. With their cancellous surfaces facing each other, the grafts are placed in the sinus tarsi with the foot held in a slightly overcorrected position.
12. As the foot is everted the grafts are locked into place, and the foot is usually so stable that if an equinus deformity is present, the tendo Achillis may be lengthened at the same operation.
13. A long leg cast is applied with the knee flexed, the ankle in maximum dorsiflexion, and the foot in the corrected position.

Grice and Green Tendon Transfer[1-5]

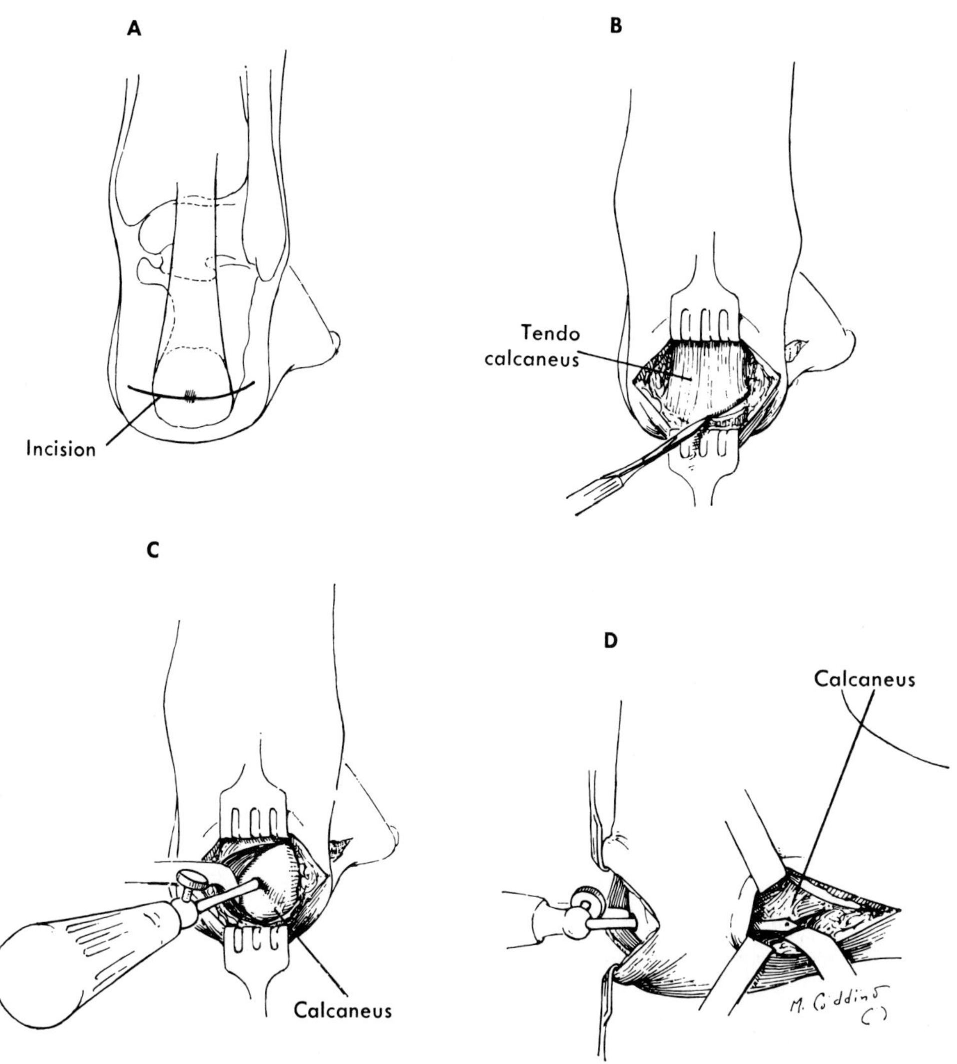

Figure 2. Green and Grice tendon transfers to calcaneus. (A) Transverse incision is made over calcaneus. (B) Beginning laterally, partially divide tendo calcaneus at its insertion. (C,D) Hole is drilled through calcaneus, beginning in center of its epiphysis and emerging at its plantar aspect near its lateral border. (E) With a twisted wire probe, tendon or tendons are brought through hole in calcaneus, and (F) are sutured to periosteum and ligamentous attachments. (G) Tendo calcaneus is sutured in its original position. (H) New course of peroneus longus muscle; peroneus brevis tendon has been sutured to distal stump of peroneus longus tendon. (Modified from Green, W.T., and Grice, D.S.: American Academy of Orthopaedic Surgeons Instructional Course Lectures, Vol. 13, J.W. Edwards, Ann Arbor, 1956. Reproduced with permission from Crenshaw, A.H. (Ed.): *Campbell's Operative Orthopaedics*, Vol. 2, C.V. Mosby, St. Louis, 1971, pp. 1576–1577.)

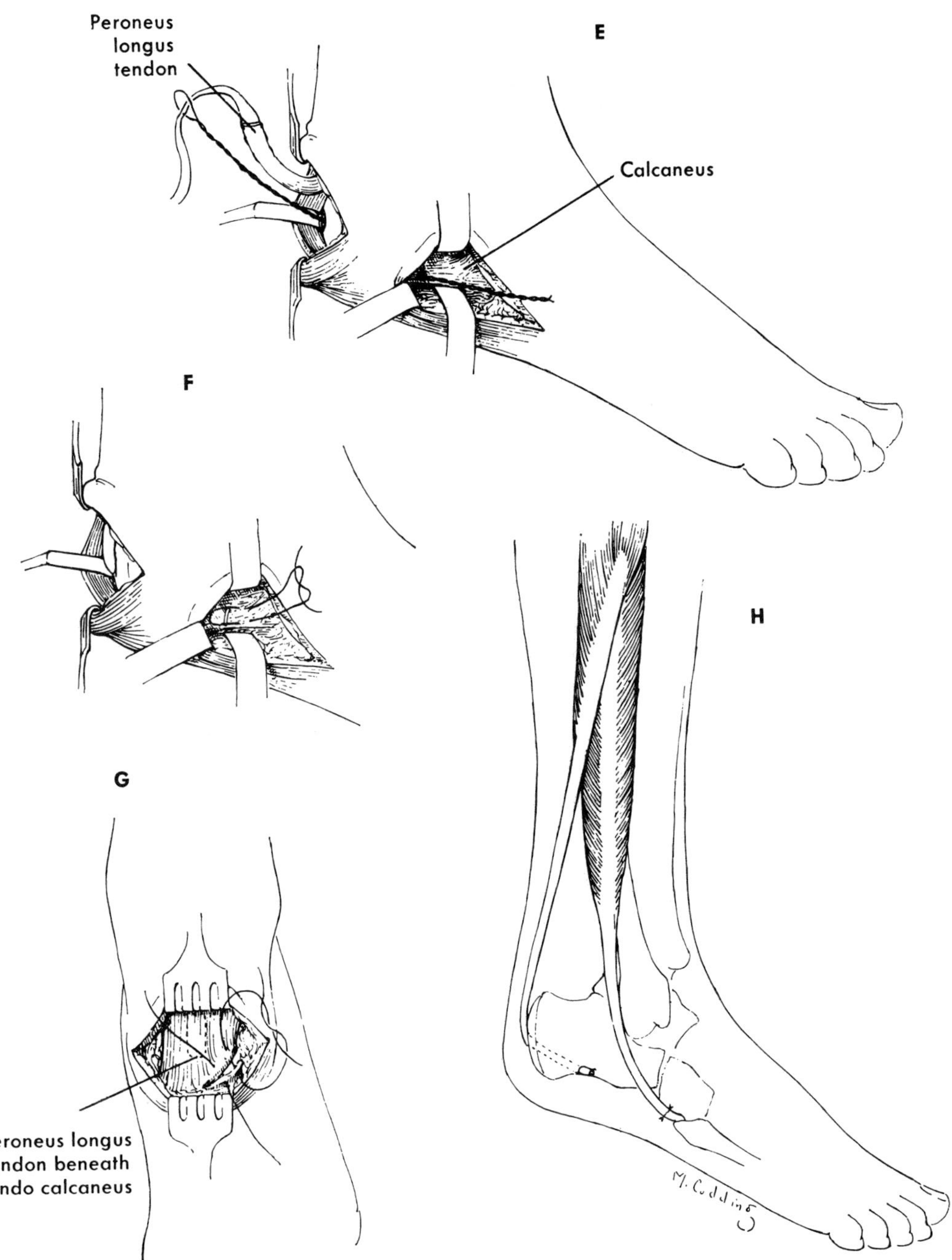

Figure 2 (continued).

1. An incision is made parallel to the bottom of the foot about a fingerbreadth distal to the lateral malleolus to the base of the fifth metatarsal.
2. The peroneus longus and brevis tendons are exposed through the length of the incision.
3. The peroneus longus is divided as far distally as possible in the sole of the

foot between two rows of sutures, and the proximal end is freed to behind the lateral malleolus.

4. A suture is then placed at the distal end of the peroneus brevis tendon just before its insertion into the base of the fifth metatarsal, and it is detached from its insertion and sutured to the distal end of the peroneus longus tendon (thereby when it contracts it will take over the function of the peroneus longus).
5. A transverse incision 6 cm long is made over the posterior aspect of the calcaneus in that part of the heel that does not strike the ground or press against the shoe (A).
6. The incision is deepened and the skin flaps are reflected subcutaneously exposing the tendo Achillis and the calcaneus.
7. Beginning laterally, partially divide the tendo Achillis at its insertion and reflect it medially to expose the calcaneal epiphysis (B).
8. With a 9/16-inch drill, make a hole through the calcaneus, beginning in the center of the epiphysis and emerging through its plantar aspect near its lateral border and into the first incision (C,D).
9. A tendon passer is inserted into the second incision and passed into the first incision, and the peroneus longus tendon is passed out of the second incision (E).
10. With a twisted wire probe passed through the hole in the calcaneus in the first incision, the tendon of the peroneus longus is brought through the hole in the calcaneus and sutured to the periosteum and ligamentous attachment where it emerges. The tendon is also sutured to the proximal end of the tunnel (F).
11. The tendo Achillis is replaced posterior to the transferred tendon and sutured in its original position (G).
12. The wound is closed in the usual manner.
13. *Modification.* The tibialis posterior and flexor longus hallucis tendons are freed through medial incisions and passed with the peroneus longus tendon through the tunnel.
14. A long leg cast is applied with the foot in equinus and the knee slightly flexed.
15. *After treatment.* Usually at three weeks the cast is bivalved and exercises are started with the leg in the anterior half of the cast. The bivalved cast is applied between exercise periods. The exercises are increased, and at six weeks the patient is allowed to stand with crutches but not to bear full weight on the foot. After six to eight weeks, a single step with crutches and an elevated heel is allowed. Steps are allowed gradually with a plantar flexion spring brace with an elastic strap posteriorly. Crutches are continued up to a year.

References

1. Green, W.T., and Grice, D.S.: The management of calcaneus deformity. *American Academy of Orthopaedic Surgeons Instructional Course Lectures*, Vol. 13, J.W. Edwards, Ann Arbor, Mich., 1956.

2. Grice, D.S.: An extra-articular arthrodesis of the subastragular joint for the correction of paralytic flat-feet in children. *J. Bone Jt. Surg.*, **34-A**:927, 1952.
3. Grice, D.S.: Further experience with extra-articular arthrodesis of the subtalar joint. *J. Bone Jt. Surg.*, **36-A**:246, 1955.
4. Grice, D.S.: The role of subtalar fusion in the treatment of valgus deformities of the feet. *American Academy of Orthopaedic Surgeons Instructional Course Lectures,* Vol. 16, C.V. Mosby, St. Louis, 1959.
5. Crenshaw, A.H. (Ed.): *Campbell's Operative Orthopaedics,* Vol. 2, C.V. Mosby, St. Louis, 1971, pp. 1563–1565, 1576–1578.

Selected Bibliography

Tachdjian, M.O.: *Pediatric Orthopaedics,* Vol. 2, W.B. Saunders, Philadelphia, 1972, pp. 804–807.

CHAPTER 11

Cavus Deformity and Clawfoot

A cavus deformity is a skeletal defect that has severe effects on joint articulation. Among the surgical procedures that have been developed to deal with the articular defects is the Steindler (calcaneal) stripping technique.[1,2] This approach does not involve arthrodesis and, alone, is insufficient to correct any but the mildest defects. Therefore, it is generally employed as a preliminary step to wrenching, osteotomy, wedge resection, or arthrodesis. Stripping, or fasciotomy, of the calcaneus is helpful because the short flexor muscles of the toes originate at the posterior process of the calcaneus, and removal of the plantar fascia relieves some of the muscle constriction. However, because muscle tissue and fascia are closely integrated, fascial stripping alone is not an adequate means of alleviating extreme contracture.

It is important to recognize that the strength of the tendo Achillis is essential to the success of surgery for correction of a cavus deformity. Therefore, if tendo Achillis lengthening is deemed necessary, this should be done as a separate procedure, either well before stripping or long enough after it that the lengthening will not affect the correction made to the cavus deformity. Without the counterforce imposed by a strong tendo Achillis, the cavus defect may redevelop.

Hibbs developed a more complex and comprehensive technique for repair of a cavus deformity.[3] In this technique also, the strength of the tendo Achillis is a critical factor. Hibbs' technique involves relieving the contracture of the plantar structures while producing a compensatory dorsiflexion by transposing the extensor digitorum longus tendon. The combined effect is a shift of power to the anterior aspect of the leg. The counterforce of the tendo Achillis against the suspended digitorum longus tendon contributes to the elimination of forefoot equinus. This procedure is not an arthrodesis unless it is combined with the Jones technique (see Chapter 9).

Another technique, one developed by Cole, involves fusion of the midtarsal bones and an anterior wedge osteotomy for cavus deformity.[4] This method has the disadvantage of shortening the dorsal surface of the foot. To obviate this negative result, Japas proposed a method by which the plantar surface of the foot is lengthened.[5] Neither of these techniques can be used to correct a cavus deformity with varus of the heel unless they are used in combination with a Dwyer osteotomy. An alternative is triple arthrodesis.

McElvenny and Caldwell devised a two-stage casting and operative procedure for correction of a cavus deformity.[6] Preliminary to the operative phase, a series of wedging casts are applied, first to place the heel in valgus, then to place the forefoot in supination. Once this has been accomplished, the cavus deformity is corrected at operation. The first metatarsal is elevated and supinated and then fused with the cuneiform. If this correction is not adequate to overcome the defect, the cuneonavicular joint is also fused.

The Dwyer technique offers three means of correcting a cavus deformity.[7-9] The closing Dwyer osteotomy is more useful in cases of persistent varus of the heel or significant pes cavus. The opening Dwyer osteotomy is used to replace the closing calcaneal osteotomy, a technique that has the disadvantage of shortening the heel. The opening procedure is ideal for correction of a cavus deformity in patients three to four years of age, but it is also useful in older children and in adolescent or adult patients with relapsed clubfoot.

The closing Dwyer osteotomy compensates for hindfoot varus in patients who are too old for Steindler stripping yet too young for triple arthrodesis.

If plantar foot contraction is significant in the patient with a cavus deformity, simultaneous removal of the plantar fascia will add to overall improvement.

A third Dwyer technique, secondary osteotomy, is also useful in cases of relapsed clubfoot. It is employed when the varus has been eliminated but the heel is small and does not touch the ground.

Steindler Stripping of the Os Calcis[2]

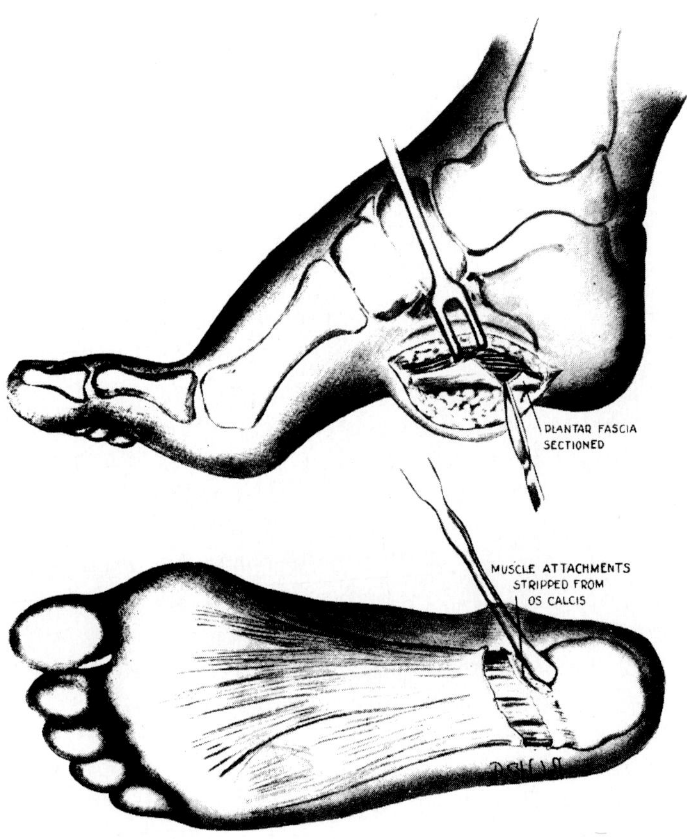

Figure 1. (Reproduced with permission from Steindler, A.: *Orthopedic Operations: Indications, Technique, and End Results,* Charles C Thomas, Springfield, Ill., 1940, p. 101.)

1. A horizontal incision is made over the inner aspect of the calcaneus forward to a point in front of the anterior process of the calcaneus.
2. The wound is deepened to the plantar fascia which is incised crosswise close to the point where it blends into the lower surface of the calcaneus.
3. The abductor hallucis, flexor brevis digitorum, and abductor minimi digiti are stripped off the periosteum of the calcaneus.
4. It is necessary to extend the stripping forward to the calcaneocuboid junction to reach and strip off the ligamentum plantare longus which extends between the calcaneus and cuboid. This ligament when contracted produces a cavity of the sole of the foot at the outer border.
5. Incision closed in the usual manner. We prefer closing the skin with subcuticular suturing using 2-0 monofilament wire.
6. *Caution*. By keeping close to the bone, one is at a safe distance from the plantar vessels and nerves. One should avoid taking along any cortical bone from the calcaneus when stripping or a great deal of bone formation may occur at the plantar surface of the calcaneus. This may be avoided by using a blunt instrument or scalpel to separate the muscles close to the periosteum.

Hibbs' Procedure[10]

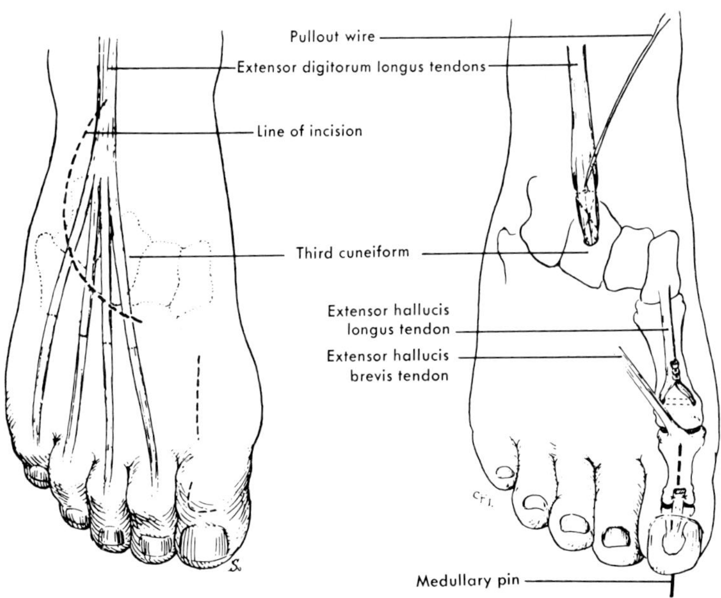

Figure 2. Hibbs operation for cavus deformity and claw foot. Tendons of extensor digitorum longus are divided, and their proximal ends are inserted as a group into third cuneiform by method of Cole. Extensor hallucis longus tendon is divided and fixed to neck of first metatarsal. Interphalangeal joint of great toe is arthrodesed and fixed with medullary pin. (Reproduced with permission from Crenshaw, A.H.: *Campbell's Operative Orthopaedics*, Vol. 2, C.V. Mosby, St. Louis, 1971, p. 1539.)

1. A Steindler stripping is performed.
   Modification. We do not omit the stripping, but McGlamry and Kitting have normally omitted the stripping and sometimes find it desirable to perform a TAL or gastrocnemius recession at the time a forefoot suspension is performed.
2. A curved longitudinal incision 3–4 inches long is made over the third cuneiform bone on the dorsum of the foot lateral to the midline and the wound deepened exposing the common extensor tendons, which are divided as far distally as possible.
   Modification. We prefer the incisions advocated by McGlamry and Kitting; i.e., a 3 cm longitudinal incision made over the second and fourth interspaces on the dorsum of the foot extending from the web proximally, and the common extensor tendons are sectioned at the level of the metatarsophalangeal joint, leaving a sufficiently long tag for attachment to the adjacent extensor digitorum brevis tendon. A third incision is made on the dorsum of the foot over the third cuneiform area, and the common extensor tendons identified and drawn proximally out of the wound and retracted.
3. A tunnel is made dorsally to plantarly through the third cuneiform bone.
4. The tips of the common extensor tendons are sutured together with either nylon or Dexon® with two Keith needles attached to the two ends of the suture, and the two needles are passed plantarly drawing the tips of the tendons of the extensor longus digitorum through the tunnel in the third cuneiform. The Keith needles are passed out through the plantar aspect of the foot, and at that point passed through a padded button and tied on the plantar surface of the foot while the foot is supported to approximately a 45 degree angle to the anterior aspect of the leg.
   Modification. The tips of the divided tendon are drawn through the tunnel in the third cuneiform and fixed with a pullout wire according to the method of Cole (see Figure 3).
5. While the foot is held in approximately a 45 degree angle to the anterior aspect of the leg, the residual distal stumps of the common extensor tendons may be anastomosed to the adjacent extensor digitorum brevis tendons, as advocated by McGlamry and Kitting.
6. Incisions are closed in the usual manner.
7. *Modifications*.
   a. If the great toe is hammered and contracted a Jones' procedure is often combined with the Hibbs' procedure.
   b. If there is a hypermobile first metatarsal segment, McGlamry and Kitting include a transposition of the extensor longus hallucis tendon into the third cuneiform bone.
   c. If there is a plantar-flexed first metatarsal segment, we perform a closing dorsal reflectory osteotomy at the base of the first metatarsal bone.
8. With the foot in the corrected position, a plaster of Paris cast is applied to the foot and leg. A walking heel is applied after two weeks and the cast worn for an additional four weeks. Physical therapy is then started and continued for an additional six weeks.

McGlamry Modification of Hibbs' Technique[11]

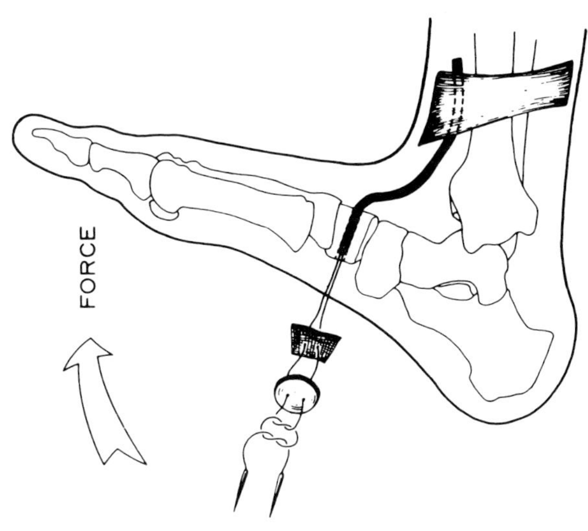

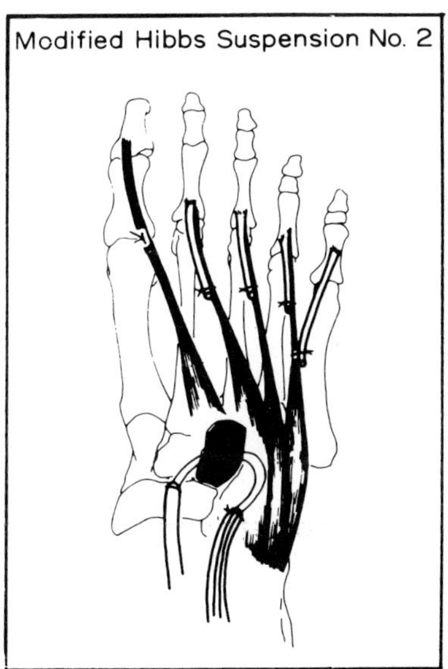

Figure 3. (Reproduced with permission from McGlamry, E.D. (Ed.): *Reconstructive Surgery of the Foot and Leg*, Intercontinental Medical Book Corporation, New York, 1974, p. 360.)

Cole Procedure

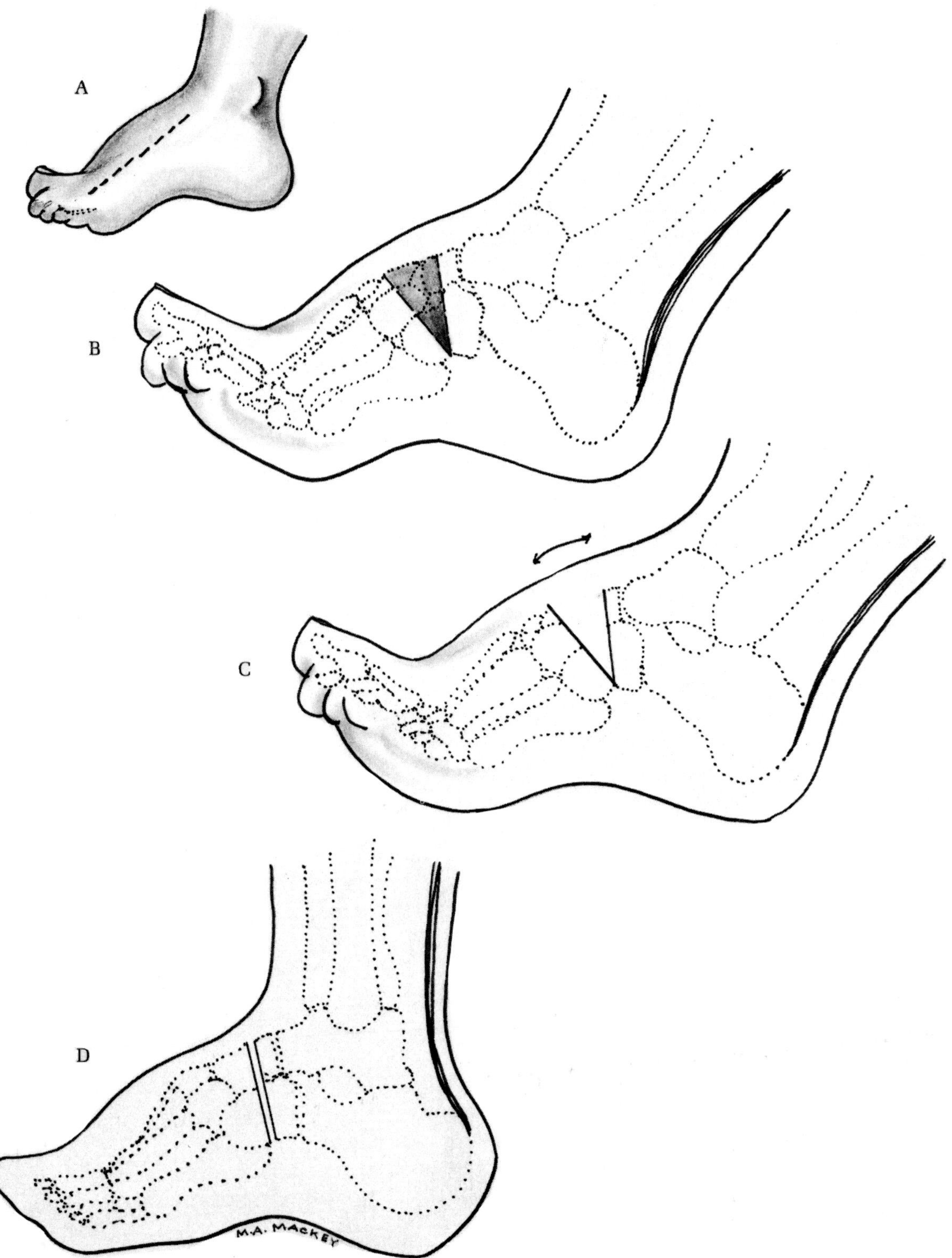

1. A Steindler stripping is performed.
2. A midline incision is made on the dorsum of the foot extending from a point just distal to the ankle joint to about the middle of the third metatarsal bone.

   Modification. Tachdjian advocates two longitudinal skin incisions. The medial incision, about 5 cm long, is over the medial aspect of the navicular and first cuneiform bones in the interval between the anterior tibial and posterior tibial tendons. The lateral incision, about 4 cm long, is centered over the cuboid bone.
3. Incised edges are undermined and retracted exposing the common extensor tendons which are retracted medially and laterally.
4. The cuneiform, navicular and cuboid bones are exposed by periosteal dissection. The capsule of the talonavicular joint should not be disturbed.
5. An almost vertical transverse osteotomy is made near the center of the navicular and cuboid to the interior surface of the tarsus.
6. A second osteotomy, beginning distal to the first and connecting with it at the inferior surface of the tarsus, is made and the wedge of bone including the navicular-cuneiform joint is excised. The distance from the proximal to the distal osteotomy (the width of the wedge) is determined by the severity of the forefoot equinus deformity to be corrected.
7. The forefoot is then manipulated into dorsiflexion to close the gap, thereby correcting the forefoot equinus. There is a dorsal displacement of the first cuneiform over the navicular in the correction. If more correction is needed, the base of the forefoot may be displaced plantarward by an osteotomy.
8. Periosteum closed with interrupted sutures.
9. *Modifications.*
   a. Tachdjian advocates fixing the osteotomy with two Steinmann pins.
   b. Meary advocates staples to fix and maintain the position of the osteotomy.
   c. At times the extensor tendons are transferred and anchored into the osteotomy site at the midline of the foot.
10. Incision is closed in the usual manner.
11. Casting and after care are similar to those for a triple arthrodesis.

Figure 4 (facing page). Cole anterior tarsal wedge osteotomy. (A) Skin incision. (B) Shaded area is wedge of bone to be excised. (C) Wedge of bone excised. (D) Osteotomy site closed, bones aligned.

Japas Procedure

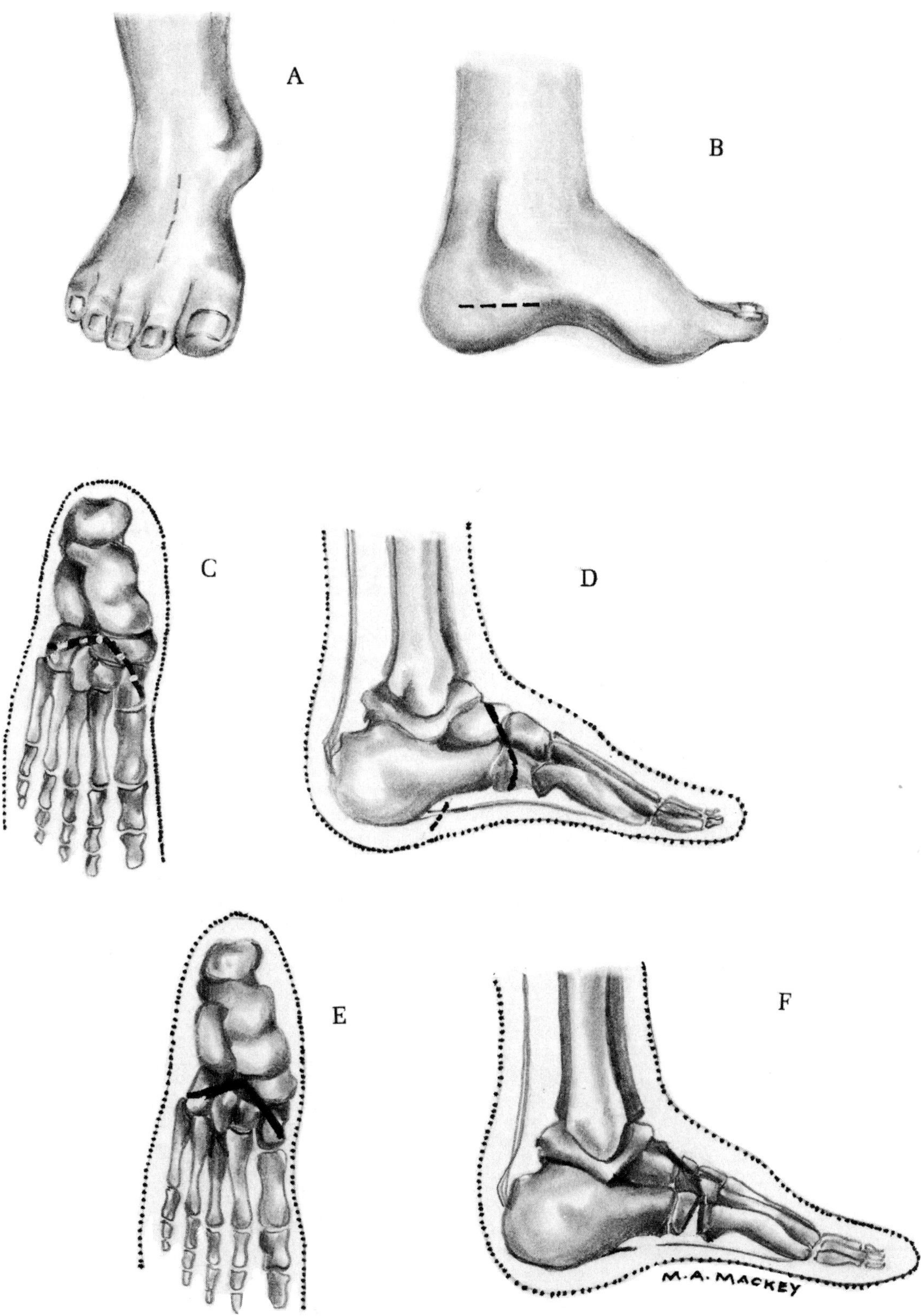

1. A Steindler plantar fasciotomy is performed.
2. A longitudinal incision approximately 6–8 cm long is made on the dorsum of the foot, extending from a midline point just distal to the ankle joint to the distal third of the third metatarsal bone.
3. Carry the dissection between the long extensor tendons of the second and third toes.
4. Retract laterally the extensor brevis digitorum and expose extraperiosteally the dorsum of the foot from the talonavicular joint to the tarsometatarsal joints.
5. With a Stryker saw a V-osteotomy is made as follows.
   a. Begin the medial limb of the osteotomy in the first cuneiform immediately proximal to the first metatarsocuneiform joint and the lateral limb in the cuboid immediately proximal to the joint between this bone and the fifth metatarsal bone.
   b. Carry these limbs proximally to join the midline of the foot at the apex of the cavus deformity, usually within the substance of the navicular. *Do not enter the midtarsal joint.*
   c. Apply traction to the distal fragment and, with the use of a periosteal elevator, depress its proximal margin plantarly while elevating the metatarsal heads.
   d. If the first metatarsal is in marked equinus, carry the medial limb of the osteotomy through the base of this bone to correct the deformity.
6. Correct any abduction or adduction deformity by simple manipulation.
7. When proper alignment has been obtained, fix the osteotomy with one or two Steinmann pins inserted in a posterior direction.
8. Incision closed in the usual manner.
9. If tendo Achillis lengthening is necessary, perform this procedure.
10. Apply a cast from the base of the toes to the tibial tuberosity.
11. Limb is elevated after surgery.
12. After two months, cast is removed and Steinmann pins are removed.
13. A walking boot is applied and worn for one month, then removed and physiotherapy started.

Figure 5 (facing page). Japas V-osteotomy of tarsus for cavus deformity. (A,B) Broken lines indicate skin incisions. (C) Osteotomy site indicated by broken line. (D) Broken lines indicate osteotomy site and Steindler stripping site. (E) Proximal margin of distal fragment depressed. (F) Steindler stripping complete. Proximal margin of distal fragment has been depressed and metatarsal heads have been elevated by opening of osteotomy site at plantar portion.

McElvenny and Caldwell Procedure[10]

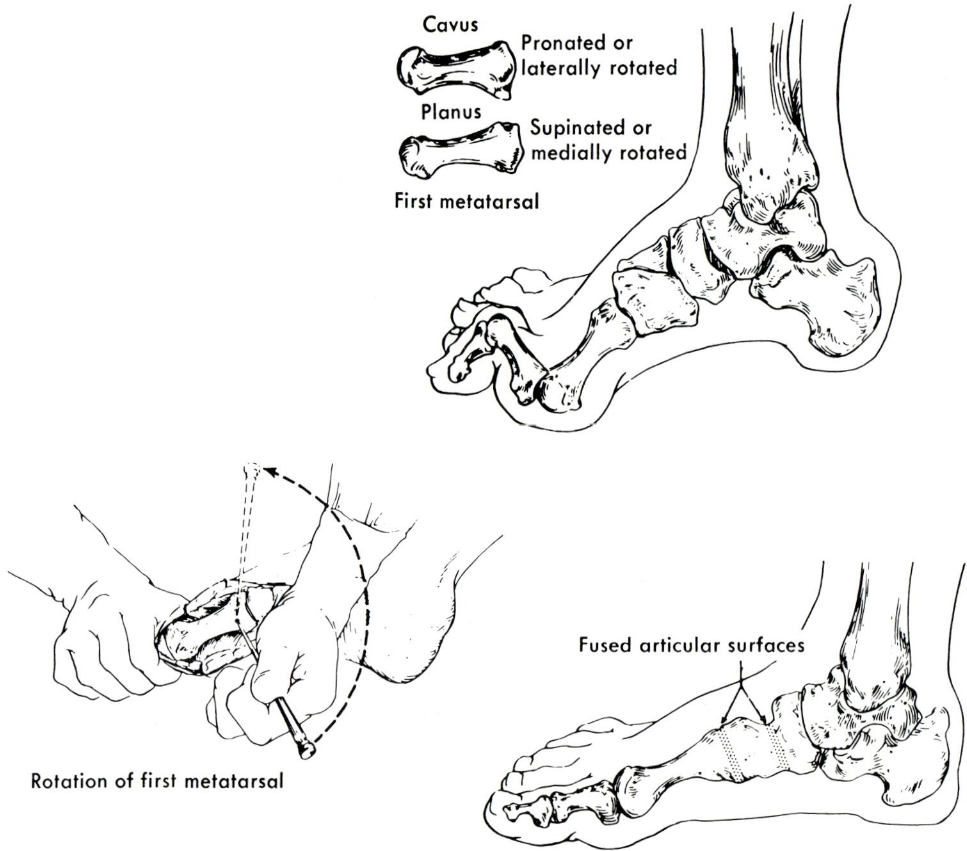

Figure 6. McElvenny and Caldwell operation that corrects cavus deformity by fusion of first metatarsocuneiform joint. Joint is denuded of cartilage and mobilized. Metatarsal is markedly supinated and its distal end is elevated; joint is then fixed with one or two threaded wires. When deformity is too severe to be competely corrected at this joint alone, naviculocuneiform joint is similarly treated. (Modified from McElvenny, R.T., and Caldwell, G.D. In A.F. DePalma (Ed.): *Clinical Orthopaedics*, Vol. 11, J.B. Lippincott, Philadelphia, 1958. Reproduced with permission from Crenshaw, A.H. (Ed.): *Campbell's Operative Orthopaedics*, Vol. 2, C.V. Mosby, St. Louis, 1971, p. 1544.)

1. Through a medial longitudinal incision, the first metatarsocuneiform joint is exposed.
2. This joint is mobilized until the first metatarsal can be elevated and supinated.
3. The cuneiform bone and the base of the first metatarsal are gradually trimmed until the desired position has been obtained and contact between these two bones is maximum.
4. Maintain the corrected position and fix the joints with one or two threaded wires. Leave the wire long enough to be incorporated into the plaster boot.

5. When the equinus of the first metatarsal is too severe to be completely corrected, the naviculocuneiform joint is denuded and trimmed until the desired correction is obtained. The position is also maintained by wire in the same manner.
6. Wound is closed in the usual manner.
7. A boot cast is applied with the forefoot in as much supination as possible and the heel in as much valgus as possible.
8. *After care.* After five weeks, the plaster is cut away exposing the wires, which are removed, and a walking heel is applied. After nine weeks the cast is removed. If x-rays show solid fusion, weight-bearing is started with an elastic bandage.

Closing Dwyer Osteotomy[12]

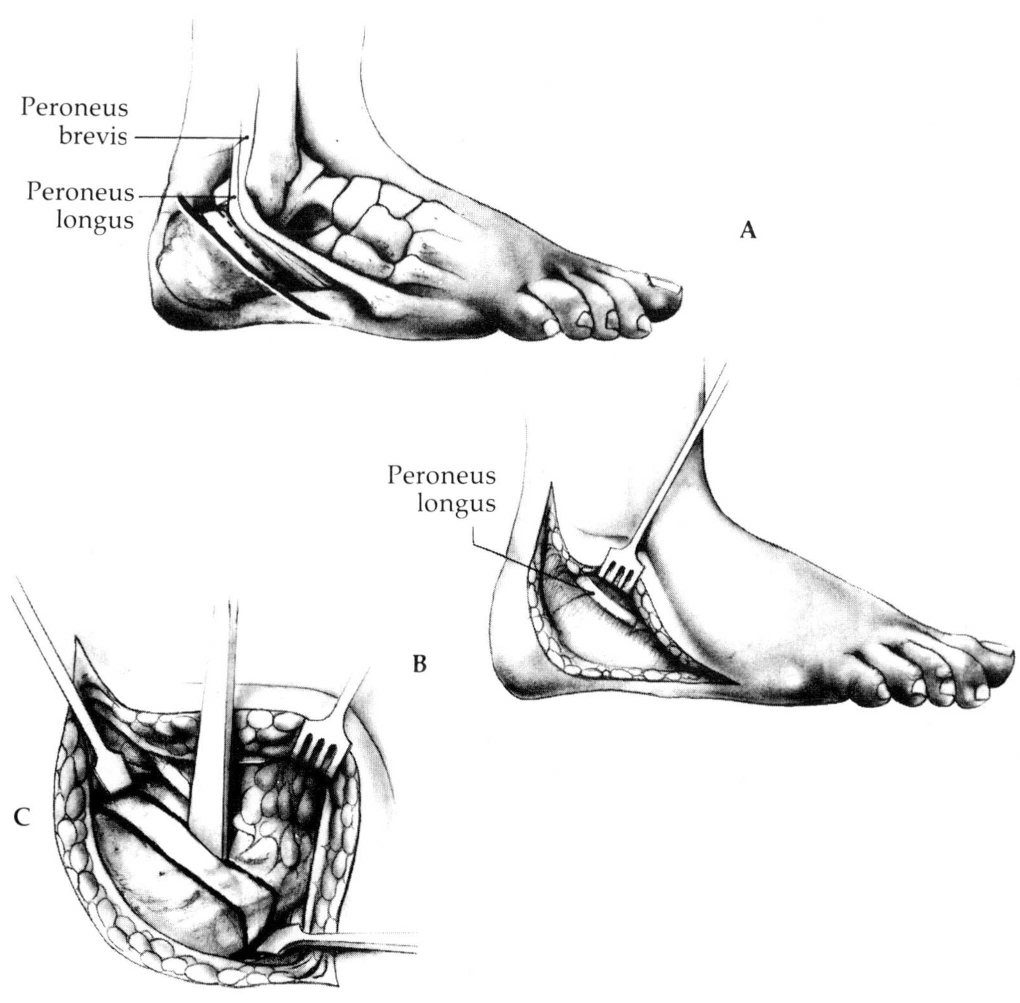

Figure 7. (Reproduced with permission from Goldstein, L.A. and Dickerson, R.C.: *Atlas of Orthopaedic Surgery,* Vol. 2, C.V. Mosby, St. Louis, 1974, pp. 905, 907.) *Continued on next page.*

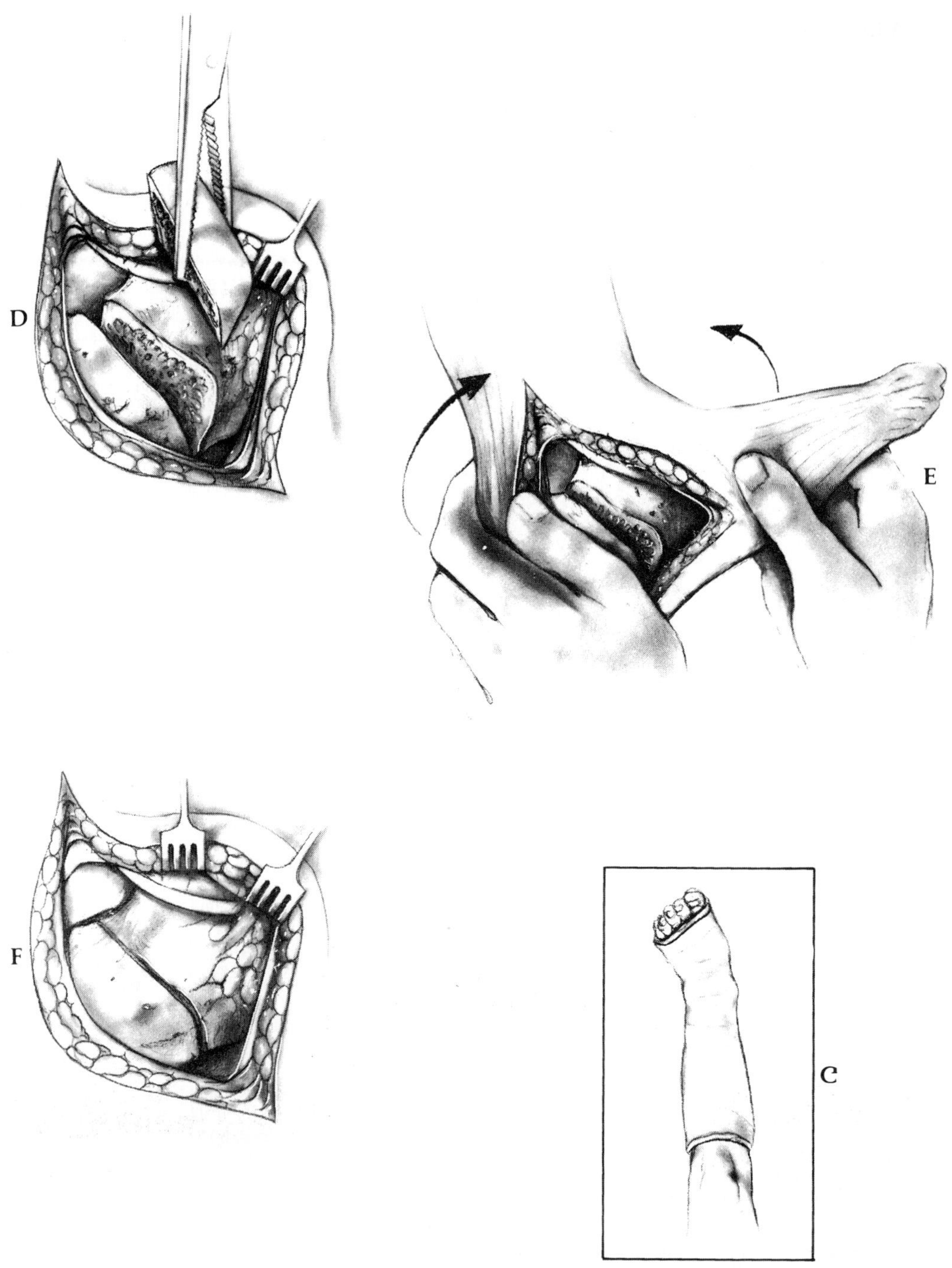

Figure 7 (continued). (Reproduced with permission from Goldstein, L.A. and Dickerson, R.C.: *Atlas of Orthopaedic Surgery,* Vol. 2, C.V. Mosby, St. Louis, 1974, pp. 905, 907.)

1. Steindler plantar fasciotomy is performed if there is significant plantar foot contracture.
2. The lateral aspect of the calcaneus is exposed through a curved incision

paralleling the peroneus longus tendon, but 1 cm posterior and inferior to it (A).

3. The entire flap is turned anteriorly until the tendon of the peroneus longus is exposed (B).
4. The periosteum is stripped from the superior, lateral and inferior surfaces of the calcaneus.
5. A wedge of bone is removed from the calcaneus just inferior and posterior to the peroneus longus tendon and parallel with it. Make the base of the wedge 8–12 mm wide and taper it without dividing the medial cortex of the calcaneus (C & D).
6. The medial cortex is broken manually to close the gap and bring the bony surfaces together by pressing the forefoot into dorsiflexion against the pull of the tendo Achillis. Failure to obtain closure is always due to a small piece of bone left behind at the apex of the wedge (E,F).
7. Make sure the varus deformity has been corrected and the heel is in a slight valgus or neutral position. Failure to correct the varus deformity completely will lead to an increase in the deformity (G).
8. Wound closed in the usual manner.
9. The foot is immobilized in a cast from the tibial tuberosity to the toes (G).
10. *After care.* Partial weight-bearing is permitted on the involved heel as soon as wound discomfort subsides. Cast is removed after the osteotomy site is united (approximately six weeks).

Opening Dwyer Osteotomy

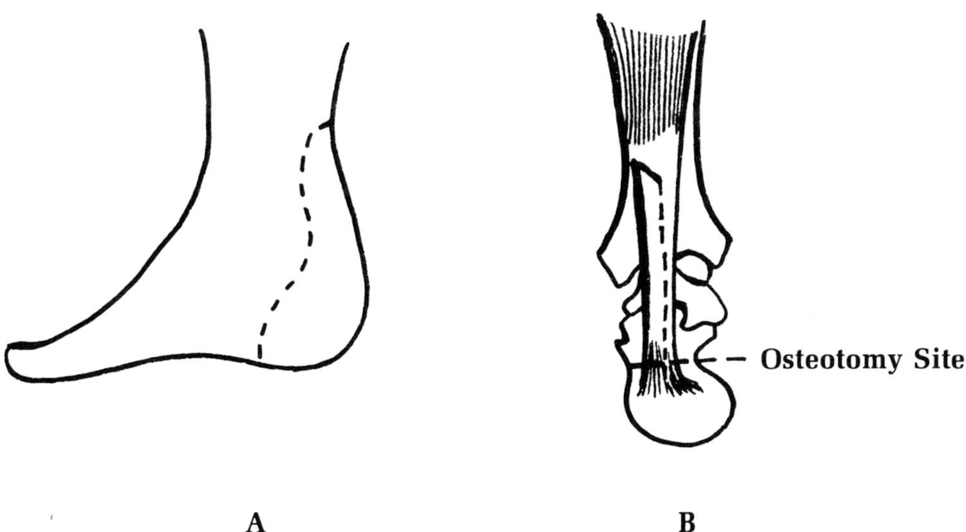

Figure 8. Dwyer osteotomy of the calcaneus for relapsed clubfoot. (A) Broken line is site of skin incision. (B) Z-plasty made into tendo Achillis, and calcaneus is osteotomized. *(Continued on next page).*

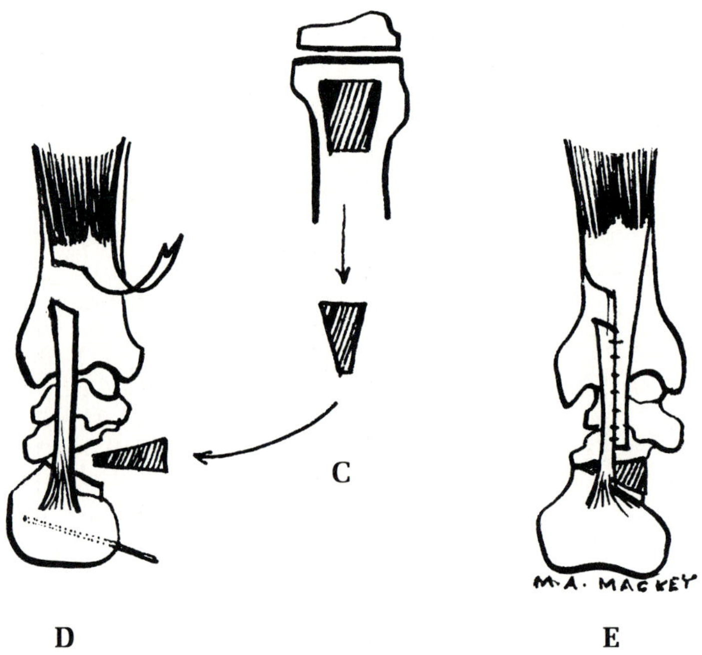

Figure 8 (continued). Dwyer osteotomy of the calcaneus for relapsed clubfoot. (C) Wedge of bone is shaped from piece of bone excised from the tibia. (D) Awl inserted into inferior fragment of calcaneus and osteotomy site is opened. (E) Wedge of bone shaped from the tibia holds open the osteotomy and the tendo Achillis is sutured in its lengthened position.

1. Expose the tendo Achillis, the heel and the plantar fascia through an incision that begins in the midline well above the heel at the level of the musculotendinous junction of the gastrosoleus, extends along the medial border of the tendo Achillis and the medial border of the heel, and ends on the sole of the foot.
2. The tendo Achillis is split in the sagittal plane and the insertion of its medial half is freed from the calcaneus.
3. The lateral half of the tendo Achillis is then divided just inferior to the musculotendinous junction.
4. On the medial side of the foot, the flexor longus hallucis tendon is exposed without damaging the neurovascular bundle.
5. The calcaneus is then divided just inferior to, and about in line with, the tendon of the flexor longus hallucis. Attempt to leave a small osteoperiosteal hinge anterolaterally.
6. Insert an awl into the inferior fragment of the bone and lever the fragment inferiorly and laterally until the deformity has been completely corrected.
7. From the proximal tibia remove a suitable wedge of bone and place it in the osteotomy. No internal fixation is necessary.
8. Remove the awl and, with the foot in full dorsiflexion, repair the tendo Achillis.
9. Carefully suture the skin beginning at the distal end of the incision pulling the anterior flap posteriorly and inferiorly with oblique sutures.
10. The foot is immobilized in a cast from the tibial tuberosity to the toes.

11. *After care.* Replace cast two weeks after surgery. Delay in healing is to be expected. Replace casts every two weeks; final cast is removed at ten weeks. Healing is usually complete at this time.

Secondary Dwyer Osteotomy[10]

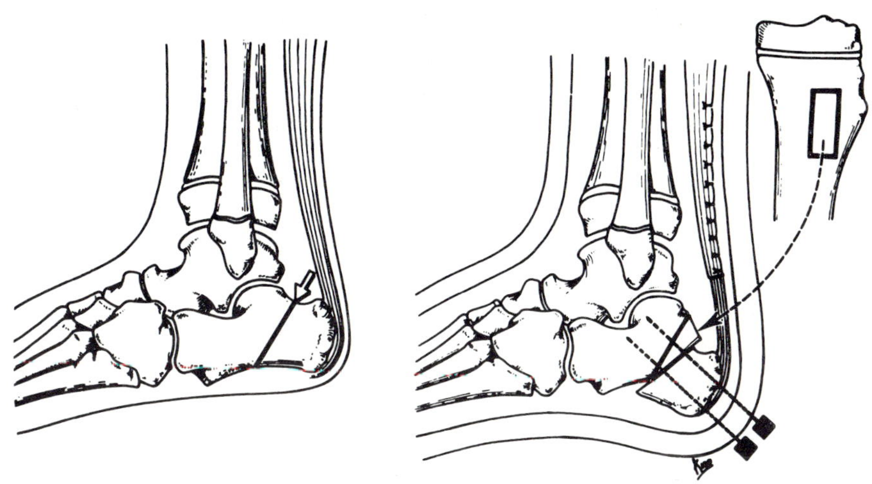

Figure 9. Secondary osteotomy of calcaneus used by Dwyer when heel is very small and fails to reach ground after varus deformity has been corrected by his usual osteotomy for relapsed clubfoot. Heel is approached from lateral side, tendo calcaneus is divided by Z-plasty, and calcaneus is osteotomized just inferior to and in line with peroneus longus tendon. Distal fragment is displaced inferiorly, suitable wedge of bone from tibia is placed in osteotomy, fragments are fixed with Kirschner wires, and tendo calcaneus is sutured. (Courtesy Mr. F.C. Dwyer. Reproduced with permission from Crenshaw, A.H.: *Campbell's Operative Orthopaedics*, Vol. 2, C.V. Mosby, St. Louis, 1971, p. 1918.)

1. Expose the tendo Achillis and the heel through an incision beginning in the midline well above the heel at the level of the musculotendinous junction of the gastrosoleus, extending along the lateral border of the tendo Achillis, and ending on the sole of the foot.
2. The tendo Achillis is divided by Z-plasty.
3. The calcaneus is osteotomized just inferior to, and in line with, the peroneus longus tendon.
4. The distal fragment is displaced inferiorly and a suitable wedge of bone is taken from the proximal tibia and placed in the osteotomy.
5. Fragments are fixed with Kirschner wires.
6. Tendo Achillis is sutured in its lengthened position with the foot in full dorsiflexion.
7. Wound is closed in the usual manner.
8. The foot is immobilized in a cast from the tibial tuberosity to the toes.
9. *After care.* Cast is removed and changed after two weeks. Kirschner wires are removed after six weeks. Final cast is removed after ten weeks.

References

1. Steindler, A.: Stripping of the os calcis. *J. Orthop. Surg.*, **2**:8, 1920.
2. Steindler, A.: *Orthopedic Operations: Indications, Technique, and End Results*, Charles C Thomas, Springfield, Ill., 1940, pp. 100–101.
3. Hibbs, R.A.: An operation for claw-foot. *J.A.M.A.*, **73**:1583, 1919.
4. Cole, W.H.: The treatment of clawfoot. *J. Bone Jt. Surg.*, **22**:895, 1940.
5. Japas, L.M.: Surgical treatment of pes cavus by tarsal v-osteotomy, preliminary report. *J. Bone Jt. Surg.*, **50-A**:927, 1968.
6. McElvenny, R.T. and Caldwell, G.D.: A new operation for the correction of cavus foot, fusion of the first metatarsocuneiform-navicular joint. In A.F. DePalma (Ed.): *Clinical Orthopaedics*, Vol. 11, J.B. Lippincott, Philadelphia, 1958.
7. Dwyer, F.C.: Osteotomy of the calcaneum for pes cavus, *J. Bone Jt. Surg.*, **41-B**:80–86, 1959.
8. Dwyer, F.C.: The treatment of relapsed club foot by the insertion of a wedge into the calcaneum. *J. Bone Jt. Surg.*, **45-B**:67–75, 1963.
9. Dwyer, F.C.: Osteotomy of the calcaneum for pes cavus. *J. Bone Jt. Surg.*, **49-B**:135, 1967.
10. Crenshaw, W.H. (Ed.): *Campbell's Operative Orthopaedics*, Vol. 2, C.V. Mosby, St. Louis, 1971, pp. 1538–1544; 1918–1919.
11. McGlamry, E.D.: *Reconstructive Surgery of the Foot and Leg*, Intercontinental Medical Book Corp., New York, 1974, pp. 358–366.
12. Goldstein, L.A., and Dickerson, R.C.: *Atlas of Orthopaedic Surgery*, Vol. 2, C.V. Mosby, St. Louis, 1974, pp. 904–907.

Selected Bibliography

Butlin, W.E.: Hibbs tendon suspension technique in the treatment of claw toe deformities, *J. of Foot Surg.*, **14**:41–44, 1975.

Inman, V.T. (Ed.): *DuVries' Surgery of the Foot*, C.V. Mosby, St. Louis, 1973, p. 493.

Larmon, W.A.: Arthrodesis of the joints of the lower extremity. *Surg. Clin. North Am.*, W.B. Saunders, Philadelphia, **1**:161–163, 1965.

Sullivan, J.D.: Calcaneal osteotomy, *J. of Foot Surg.*, **16**:17–23, 1977.

Tachdjian, M.: *Pediatric Orthopedics*, Vol. II, W.B. Saunders, 1972.

Wolff, L.J.: Review of treatment and diagnosis of pes cavus and associated abnormalities. *Arch. of Pod. Med. & Foot Surg.*, **2**:121–131, 1974.

CHAPTER 12

Longitudinal Arch Correction

Various surgical techniques for longitudinal arch correction to overcome a flatfoot deformity have been developed for children, adolescents, and adults. The Kidner procedure is ideal for children with the type of flatfoot characterized by an accessory navicular.[1,2] Most often this condition involves incorrect attachment of the tibialis posterior tendon to the accessory bone, from which it passes above the medial aspect of the navicular rather than below it. When this situation is present, longitudinal arch support is lost. In some instances, the medial aspect of the navicular is enlarged and curved in such a way that the tendon of the tibialis posterior is abnormally inserted. Correction of the mechanical defect in either case is the same. Lengthening of the tendo Achillis may also be indicated.

Two other techniques, those devised by Miller[3] and by Hoke,[4,5] require preoperative roentgenograms to determine whether the deformity is in the cuneonavicular joint or in the talonavicular joint. If a sag in the talonavicular is overlooked, the correction obtained by either technique will be threatened. Furthermore, in a foot with a fixed valgus deformity, excessive relaxation of the major joints of the foot, or any tarsal defect, these procedures are not indicated at all.

The Lowman[6] procedure was developed to correct flatfoot when the primary cause of the defect is a long talar neck. The technique involves resection of the talar head, displacement of the tibialis anterior tendon, and arthrodesis of the talonavicular joint. This approach is best suited to adults with rigid pes planus and normal peroneals and to adolescents with flexible pes planus from sag at the talonavicular joint.

A modification of Lowman's procedure was devised by Young[7] to correct defects in patients over the age of ten. It can be used when the major tarsal joints are not involved. With this modification, the tibialis anterior muscle is transferred to serve as an active arch elevator. In the transfer, the tibialis anterior tendon also is displaced into a position inferior to the navicular and cuneiform, where it provides added ligamentous support to the arch.

Kidner Procedure[8]

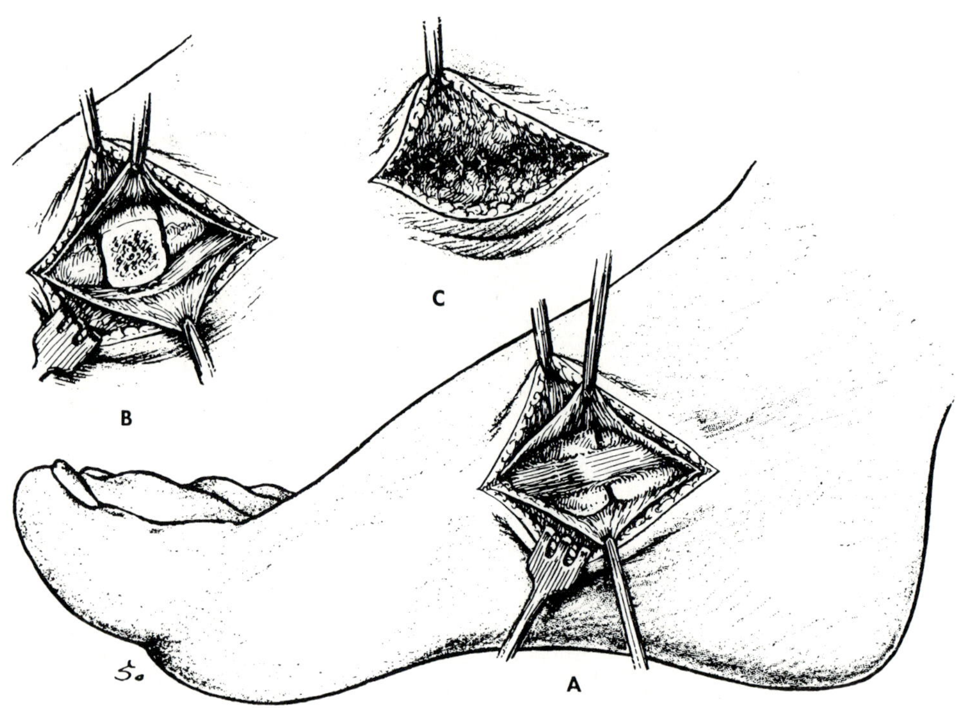

Figure 1. Kidner operation for pes planus with accessory navicular (prehallux). (A) Approach exposes tibialis posterior tendon and accessory navicular. (B) Tibialis posterior tendon along with small fragment of bone has been freed from navicular and transposed inferiorly. Accessory navicular and medial surface of navicular have been excised. (C) Closure. (Reproduced with permission from Crenshaw, A.H. (Ed.): *Campbell's Operative Orthopaedics*, Vol. 2, C.V. Mosby, St. Louis, 1971, p. 1798.)

1. Begin the incision inferior to the medial malleolus, curve it slightly plantarly and extend it distally to the base of the first metatarsal.
2. Incise the fascia and periosteum longitudinally.
3. Free the uppermost dorsal insertions of the tibialis posterior preserving its attachment to the accessory navicular and to the plantar surface of the cuneiforms.
4. Elevate the fascia and periosteum from the inferior and superior surfaces of the navicular and of the head and neck of the talus, making dorsal and plantar flaps.
5. With a thin osteotome free the tibialis posterior tendon with a small fragment of bone from the tuberosity of the navicular.
6. Detach the medial fibers of the tendon from the first cuneiform, but leave the inferior distal fibers undisturbed.
7. Transpose the tendon plantarly and laterally into a groove on the plantar surface of the navicular. Usually a groove is present; if not, create one with an osteotome.

8. Then remove the accessory navicular and resect the medial aspect of the navicular until it is flush with the talus and cuneiform.
9. Holding the tendon under slight tension and the foot in moderate cavus and supination, fasten the tendon to the plantar flap of the fascia and periosteum as far laterally on its plantar fascia as possible with chromic catgut. If the plantar flap is not strong fasten tendon by passing the sutures through two holes drilled plantarly through the middle of the navicular.
10. Suture the dorsal and plantar flaps of fascia and periosteum over the raw surface of the navicular and bury the tendon in its new bed.
11. Incision is closed in the usual manner.
12. The cast is applied in two sections. The first encases only the foot, with the foot in equinus and the heel in varus. After the cast has hardened, the ankle is dorsiflexed to neutral and more plaster is applied to make a long leg cast with the knee in slight flexion.
13. After two weeks, the cast and sutures are removed and a boot cast is applied and worn for four weeks. Then a walking boot cast is applied for four more weeks. Thereafter a sturdy shoe with orthoses should be worn for several months.

Miller Procedure

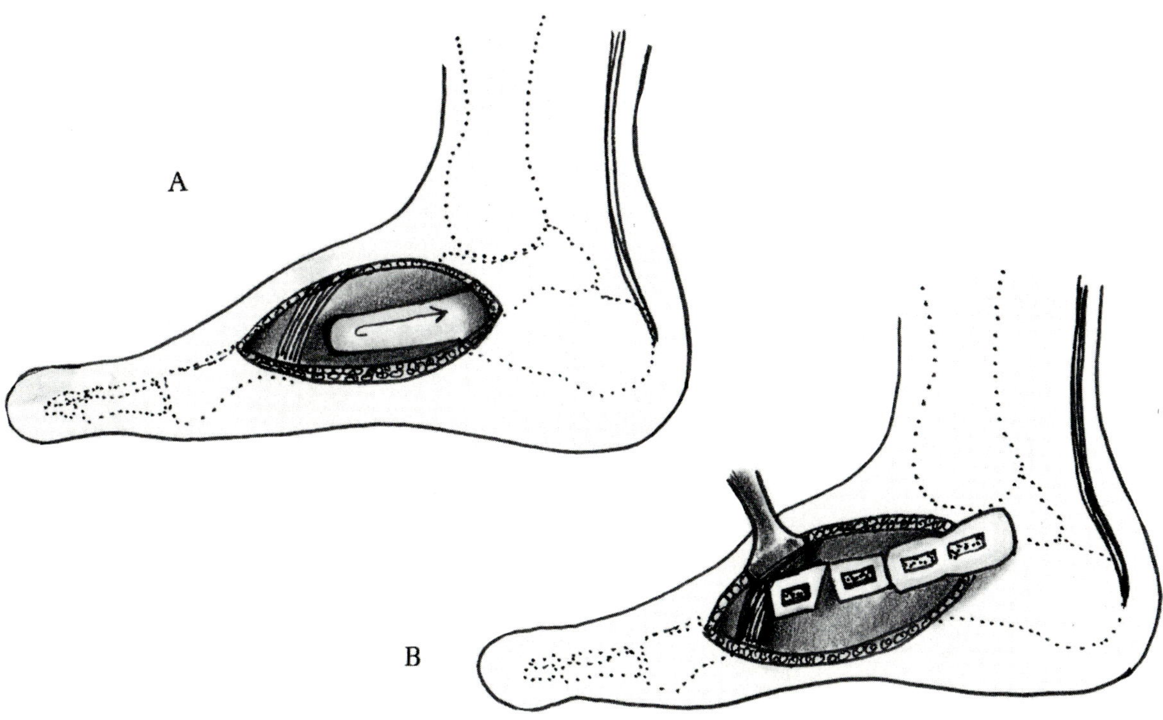

Figure 2. Miller procedure for flexible pes planus. (A) U-incision made on medial aspect of talonavicular, navicular-cuneiform, and first metatarsocuneiform joints. (B) Strip raised and reflected proximally. *(Continued on next page)*.

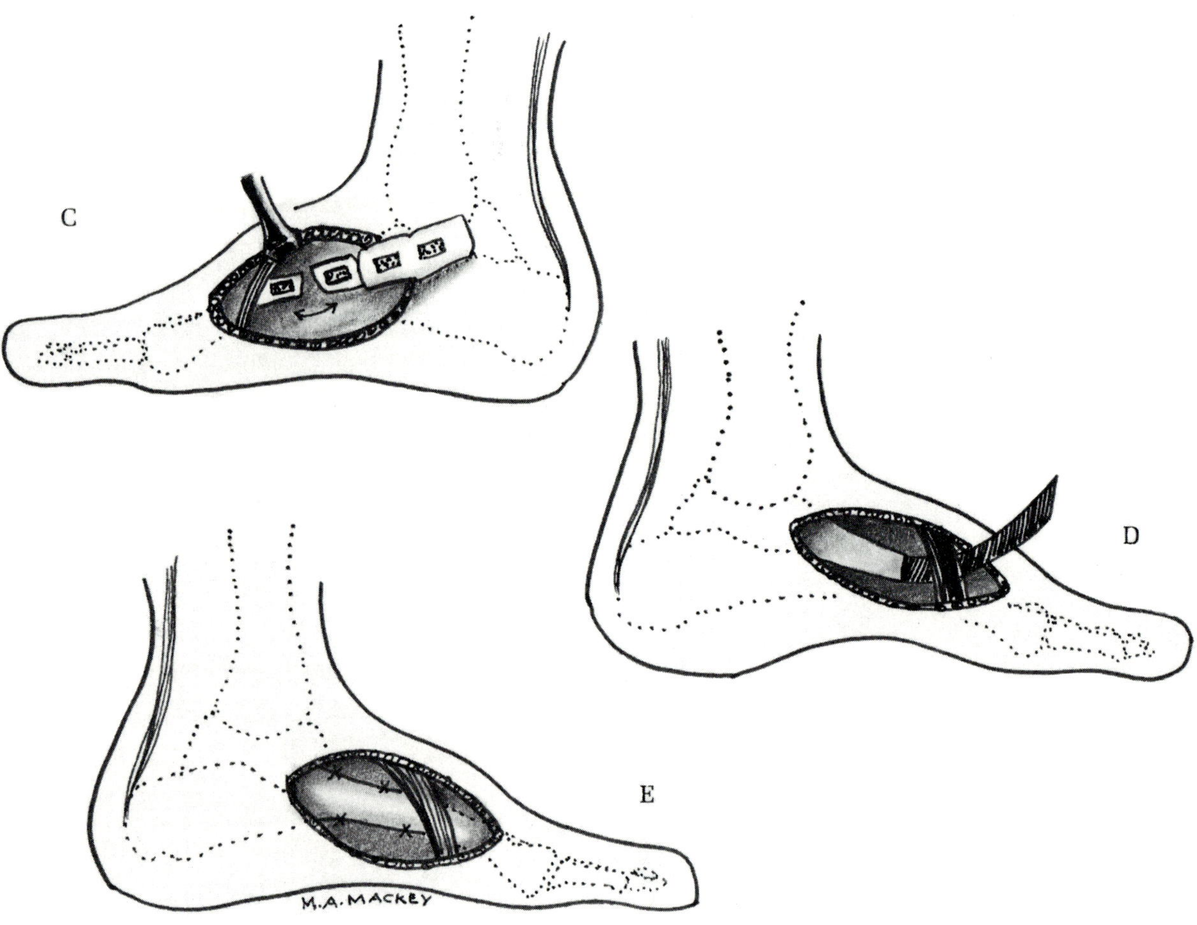

Figure 2 (continued). Miller procedure for flexible pes planus. (C) Wedge of bone removed from navicular-cuneiform joint. (D,E) Deformity reduced with flap pulled distally and sutured under tension.

1. Lengthen the tendo Achillis if indicated.
2. Along the medial side of the foot make a gently curved incision, convex dorsally, beginning at the calcaneus, proceeding distally across the navicular and first cuneiform, and ending at the base of the first metatarsal.
3. Wound edges undermined and retracted exposing the plantar calcaneonavicular ligament and the insertion of the tibialis anterior and posterior.
4. Define and elevate the tendon of the tibialis anterior.
5. Then with a sharp thin osteotome, raise with its base proximally a strip about 5/8 inch wide consisting of (1) the fanned-out insertions of the plantar calcaneonavicular ligament and the tibialis posterior tendon, and (2) thin slabs of underlying bone from the medial aspect of the navicular and the first cuneiform.

6. The strip is reflected proximally exposing the talonavicular, navicular-cuneiform and the first metatarsocuneiform joints.
7. Reflect dorsally and plantarly the lesser articular ligaments.
8. Remove the articular cartilage and subchondral bone from the naviculocuneiform and first metatarsocuneiform joints in wedges of appropriate size to correct the pes planus. Roughen the raw osseous surfaces to ensure fusion.
9. Should the navicular be prominent medially, resect the protruding bone.
10. Pull distally the strip of tissue that had been raised consisting of tendon, ligament and bone, slipping it beneath the tibialis anterior tendon, and suture it under tension to the first cuneiform and the base of the first metatarsal, thereby advancing the insertion of both tendon and ligament.
11. Suture the fascia in place and close the wound in the usual manner.
12. Casting and after care are the same as for the Kidner operation.

Hoke's Procedure

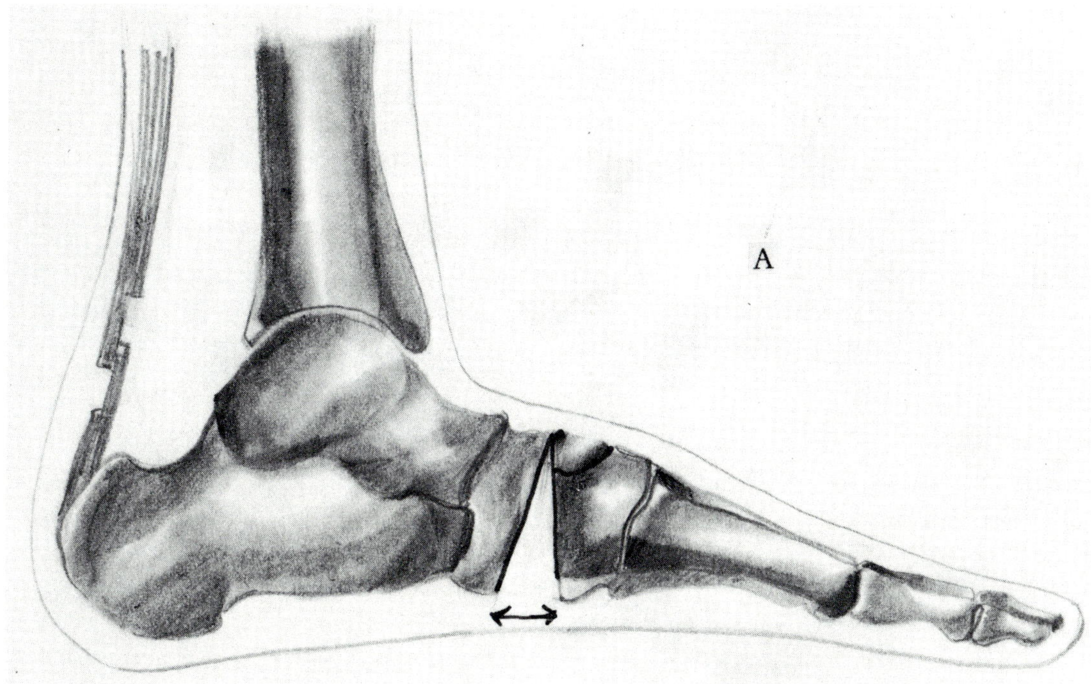

Figure 3. Hoke procedure for flexible pes planus. (A) Tendo Achillis lengthened. The articular cartilage from the opposing surfaces of the navicular and the first and second cuneiforms are excised in a wedge-shaped fashion. *(Continued on next page.)*

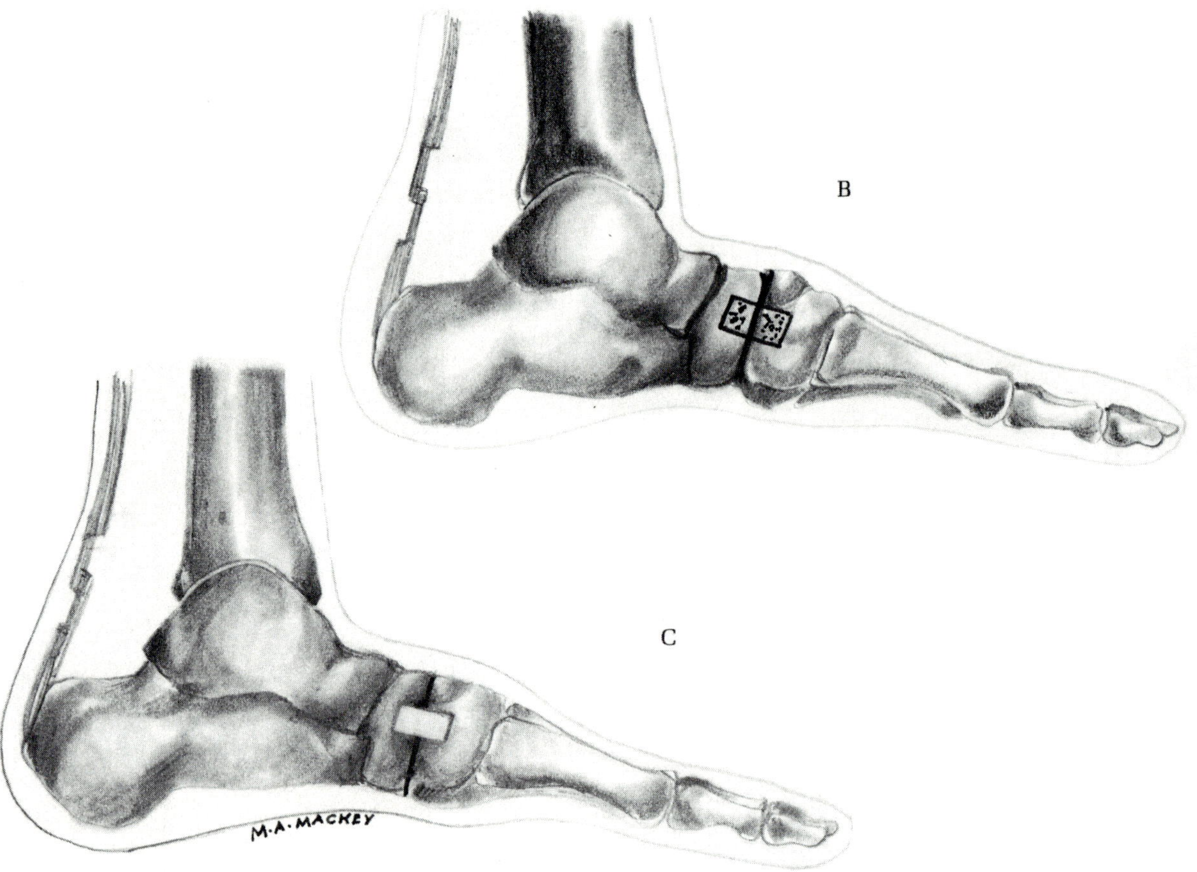

Figure 3 (continued). (B) Foot and distal end of first metatarsal are forced into equinus. A rectangular block of bone is excised from the navicular and first cuneiform across the joint. (C) A piece of cortical bone from the tibia is fitted as an inlay graft to bridge the joint.

1. Lengthen the tendo Achillis if indicated.
2. Make an incision along the medial border of the foot to expose the naviculocuneiform joint.
3. Excise the articular cartilage from the opposing surfaces of the navicular and the first and second cuneiforms.
4. Force the foot and the distal end of the first metatarsal into equinus and, while holding them in this position, resect a rectangular block of bone from the navicular and first cuneiform across the joint.
5. Then remove from the tibia a piece of cortical bone the same size as the block of bone resected from the navicular and first cuneiform and fit it in as an inlay graft into the rectangular gap to bridge the joint.
6. Pack small fragments of bone into any unfilled spaces and close the soft tissues over the graft.
7. Close the wound in the usual manner.
8. Casting and after care are the same as for the Kidner operation.

Lowman's Procedure[8]

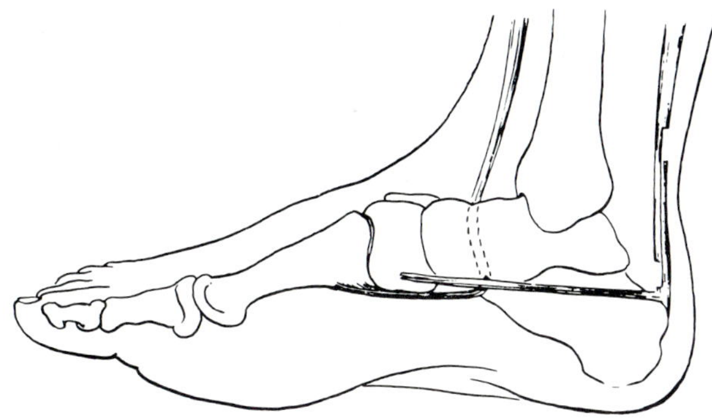

Figure 4. Lowman operation for pes planus. Note that talonavicular joint is arthrodesed, including transposed tibialis anterior tendon. Tendo calcaneus is lengthened by Z-plasty, strip of tendon being brought forward as new ligament to maintain calcaneus and forefoot in adduction. (Reproduced with permission from Crenshaw, A.H. (Ed.): *Campbell's Operative Orthopaedics*, Vol. 2, C.V. Mosby, St. Louis, 1971, p. 1802.)

1. A straight posterior skin incision is made medial to the tendo Achillis.
2. Skin edges undermined and retracted exposing the sheath of the tendo Achillis, which is opened longitudinally.
3. A strip of tendon ¼ inch wide and 5 inches long is dissected from the medial border of the tendo Achillis. If the plantaris tendon is present, use it instead.
4. The tendo Achillis is lengthened by Z-plasty to allow the foot when inverted to dorsiflex 5 degrees.
5. Make a second longitudinal incision, convex dorsally, on the medial border of the foot, beginning it inferior to the medial malleolus and extending it to a point dorsal to the navicular and then distally and plantarly to the medial side of the base of the first metatarsal.
6. Incise the fascia in a straight line to expose the tuberosity of the navicular and the medial side of the plantar calcaneonavicular ligament.
7. Divide the talonavicular ligament in line with the talonavicular joint and expose subperiosteally the medial aspect of the navicular.
8. Remove from the talonavicular joint a wedge of bone, the base of which is medial and plantar. Excise enough bone from the head of the talus to allow full correction of the abnormal abduction of the forefoot and the flatness of the longitudinal arch.
9. Free the tibialis anterior tendon distally to its insertion, and retract it medially and plantarly until it slips over the corner of the navicular into the space created by the osteotomy.
10. Displace the tendon between the talus and the navicular as far laterally as possible so that its pull will elevate the apex of the longitudinal arch, firmly suture the plantar calcaneonavicular ligament to the tendon and overlap and suture the cut ends of the talonavicuar ligament, thereby, in effect, shortening the calcaneonavicular ligament.

11. Now, subcutaneously draw the previously dissected slip of the tendo Achillis or the tendon of the plantaris into the medial incision and suture it to that segment of the tibialis anterior tendon which lies on the plantar surface of the navicular. This slip of tendon maintains both the calcaneus and forefoot in adduction and reinforces the calcaneonavicular ligament.
12. Incisions closed in the usual manner.
13. With the foot in the corrected position and the knee in slight flexion, a cast is applied from just proximal to the knee to the base of the toes.
14. After four weeks the cast is removed and a walking boot cast is applied. Weight-bearing is permitted in eight weeks. After 3 months, the second cast is removed and shoes with rigid orthoses are fitted and worn for one year.

Young's Procedure[8]

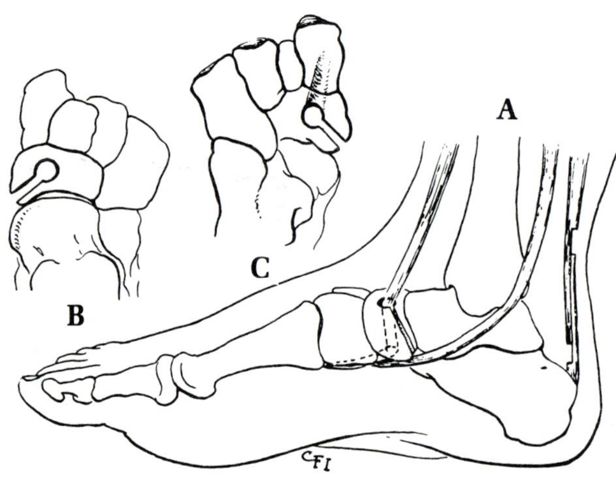

Figure 5. Young operation for pes planus. (A) Tibialis anterior tendon is translocated into slot in navicular, and tendo calcaneus is lengthened if necessary. (B,C) Note location of slot in navicular. (Reproduced with permission from Crenshaw, A.H. (Ed.): *Campbell's Operative Orthopaedics*, Vol. 2, C.V. Mosby, St. Louis, 1971, p. 1802.)

1. Lengthen the tendo Achillis if indicated.
2. Incision is made on the medial side of the foot as in the Lowman operation.
3. Dissect the tibialis posterior tendon from its insertion.
4. Drill a hole ¼ inch in diameter plantarly through the navicular, ½ inch lateral to its tuberosity.
5. Gouge the dorsal opening of the hole to make it ovoid.
6. Make a groove in the plantar surface of the first cuneiform and the navicular from the insertion of the tibialis anterior tendon to the hole just drilled.
7. Make a slot 3/16 inch wide connecting the hole with the posteromedial angle of the tuberosity of the navicular.

8. Open the distal 2½ inches of the sheath of the tibialis anterior tendon and free the tendon down its insertion to avoid later tension on the soft parts when weight is borne.
9. Pull the tendon posteriorly and make it pass through the slot in the navicular.
10. Fill the slot with bone chips.
11. Reattach the tibialis posterior tendon with interrupted sutures.
12. Incision is closed in the usual manner.
13. If the tendo Achillis has been lengthened, a long leg cast is applied that holds the ankle dorsiflexed 5 degrees and the knee flexed 20 degrees.
14. The cast is windowed and the sutures are removed in two weeks. All immobilization is discontinued after eight weeks. Walking is not permitted until then.
15. If the tendo Achillis has not been lengthened, a short leg cast is applied. After four weeks the cast is altered for walking.

References

1. Kidner, F.C.: The pre hallux (accessory scaphoid) in its relation to flat foot. *J. Bone Jt. Surg.*, **11**:831, 1921.
2. Kidner, F.C.: The pre hallux in relation to flat foot. *J.A.M.A.*, **101**:1539, 1933.
3. Miller, O.L.: A plastic flatfoot operation. *J. Bone Jt. Surg.*, **9**:84, 1927.
4. Hoke, M.J.: An operation for the correction of extremely relaxed flat feet. *J. Bone Jt. Surg.*, **13**:772–773, 1931.
5. Hoke, M.J.: An operation for stabilizing paralytic feet. *Am. J. Orthoped. Surg.*, **3**:494, 1921.
6. Lowman, C.L.: An operative method for correction of certain forms of flat foot. *J.A.M.A.*, **101**:1539, 1933.
7. Young, C.S.: Operative treatment of pes planus. Surg. *Gynecol. Obstet.*, **68**:1099, 1939.
8. Crenshaw, A.H. (Ed.): *Campbell's Operative Orthopaedics*, Vol. 2, C.V. Mosby, St. Louis, 1971, pp. 1797–1803.

Selected Bibliography

Frankel, J.P.: Surgical considerations for correction of flatfoot deformity. *J. of Foot Surg.*, **14**:81–91, 1975.

Larmon, W.A.:O Arthrodesis of the joints of the lower extremity. Surg. *Clin. North Am.*, W.B. Saunders, Philadelphia, **1**:163–165, 1965.

Subotnick, S.I.: The flexible flatfoot. *Arch. of Pod. Med. & Foot Surg.*, **1**:7–34, 1973.

CHAPTER 13

Rocker Bottom Flatfoot

Congenital convex pes valgus, also known as rocker bottom flatfoot or vertical talus flatfoot, is characterized by dislocation of the talonavicular joint, which has the effect of locking the joint so that the calcaneus is everted in a rigid, plantar-flexed position and the foot is in extreme equinus. This defect also causes curvature of the medial and plantar surfaces of the foot, which gives the rocker bottom appearance to the sole. At the midtarsal joint dorsiflexion and abduction of the forefoot pull the navicular over the dorsal edge of the talar heel. The net effect is a fixed calcaneovalgus deformity of the forefoot in combination with equinovalgus of the hindfoot.

There does not appear to be a hereditary factor in rocker bottom flatfoot as in congenital talipes calcaneovalgus. Rocker bottom flatfoot has been seen as a manifestation of the Ehlers-Danlos Syndrome. Mau[1] feels that a spinal cord lesion in early embryonic life with a muscle imbalance causes the peroneal muscles to be stronger than the invertors of the foot with the formation of a secondary congenital rigid flatfoot. Many authors have reported that they have noted a high percentage of neurological disorders associated with this foot deformity. It has been concluded that rocker bottom flatfoot is probably a deformity of congenital origin occurring approximately 50 percent of the time with other congenital birth defects or endocrine disturbances such as hypopituitarism. Rocker bottom flatfoot may very rarely exhibit an hereditary pattern.

In early infancy congenital convex pes valgus must be differentiated from talipes calcaneovalgus, which also is characterized by forefoot dorsiflexion and eversion and by limited plantar flexion of the hindfoot. The differential diagnosis is made on the basis of presence or absence of the plantar convexity and the extreme rigidity characteristic of rocker bottom flatfoot.

Treatment of the congenital defect is begun early, with serial casting and closed reduction. These conservative measures should be employed for three months, and if they fail to effect a correction the patient must undergo operation. With development, abduction of the foot with convex pes valgus causes weightbearing to center on the talus, which then becomes misshapen until talar articulation with the tibia is all but lost. Operative techniques developed by Ingram[2], by Hark[3], and by Herndon and Heyman[4] are directed at restoration of tarsal articulation by means of soft tissue repairs. Choice of operative technique is dictated by patient age and the nature and degree of the defect. In patients under the age of ten, muscle and tendon contractures are repaired; if this correction is insufficient, extra-articular arthrodesis will then be necessary. For patients over the age of ten, the correction of tissue contracture must be combined with triple arthrodesis.

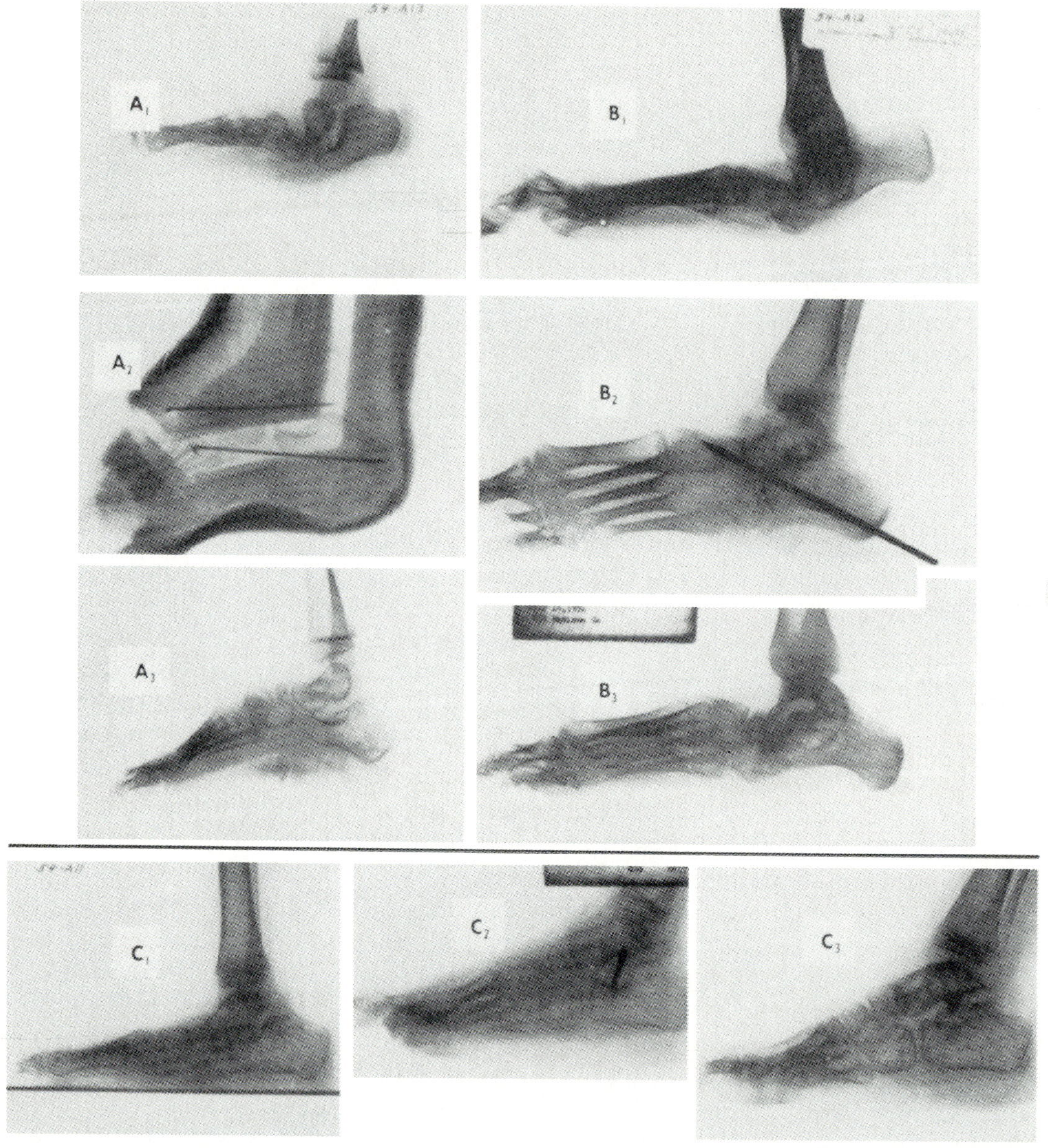

Figure 1. Surgical treatment of congenital rocker bottom flatfoot. (A_1) Severe deformity before surgery. (A_2) Lateral roentgenogram made immediately after surgery shows that deformity has been corrected and that tarsals have been fixed internally with Kirschner wires. Corrected position has been maintained even though cast has been bivalved. (A_3) Early result is excellent, but later if deformity tends to recur, extra-articular arthrodesis (Grice) will be required. (B_1) Severe deformity before surgery. (B_2) Fairly satisfactory position after surgery. (B_3) Deformity recurred within nine months after surgery. Triple arthrodesis is now required. (C_1) Deformity before surgery. (C_2) After deformity has been corrected surgically and subtalar joint fused extra-articularly (Grice). (C_3) Excellent result two years after surgery. (Reproduced with permission from Crenshaw, A.H. (Ed.): *Campbell's Operative Orthopaedics*, Vol. 2, C.V. Mosby, St. Louis, 1971, p. 1923.)

Ingram Procedure[5]

1. Make medial and lateral incisions as in releasing operations for resistant clubfoot.
2. Through the medial incision, free the soft tissue structures around the talonavicular joint, the medial aspect of the subtalar joint, and the posterior aspect of the ankle joint.
3. Through the lateral incisions free the structures around the lateral aspect of the calcaneocuboid and subtalar joints.
4. Lengthen the peroneus brevis tendon by Z-plasty, and place the talus in position to articulate with the navicular.
5. Dislocate the talonavicular joint and pass a Kirschner wire posteriorly through the head, neck, and body of the talus to emerge on the posterior aspect of the foot.
6. Reduce the joint and drill the wire distally through the navicular, the first cuneiform and the base of the first metatarsal so that it emerges through the dorsum of the foot. Advance the wire until its posterior end is at the posterior aspect of the talus.
7. Lengthen the tendo Achillis by Z-plasty; place the calcaneus in its normal position and fix with Kirschner wire through the calcaneocuboid joint.
8. Divide the posterior tibial tendon at its insertion and suture it to the periosteum inferior to the talar neck.
9. Free the tibialis anterior tendon and suture it to the posterior tibial tendon.
10. With the foot in position, apply a long leg cast, which will be worn for six to eight weeks.

Hark Procedure[3]

1. Lengthen the tendo Achillis by Z-plasty.
2. Insert a Steinmann pin transversely across the posterior superior surface of the calcaneus to hold it in the calcaneus position.
3. Expose the midtarsal area with two incisions: (a) anterolaterally over the sinus tarsus and (b) medially to the tibialis anterior tendon.
4. Lengthen the tibialis anterior and extensor hallucis longus tendons by Z-plasty.
5. Divide the extensor digitorum tendons, cutting two alternate tendons and the proximal and distal ends.
6. Correct midtarsal dislocation by capsulotomies of the talonavicular and calcaneocuboid joints.
7. Join the extensor tendons by suturing the long ends to each other and the short ends to the sides of the long ends, thus converting four short tendons into two long ones.
8. Transfix the midtarsal joint with Kirschner wires and cast for six to eight weeks.

Herndon and Heyman Procedure for Correction of Vertical Talus

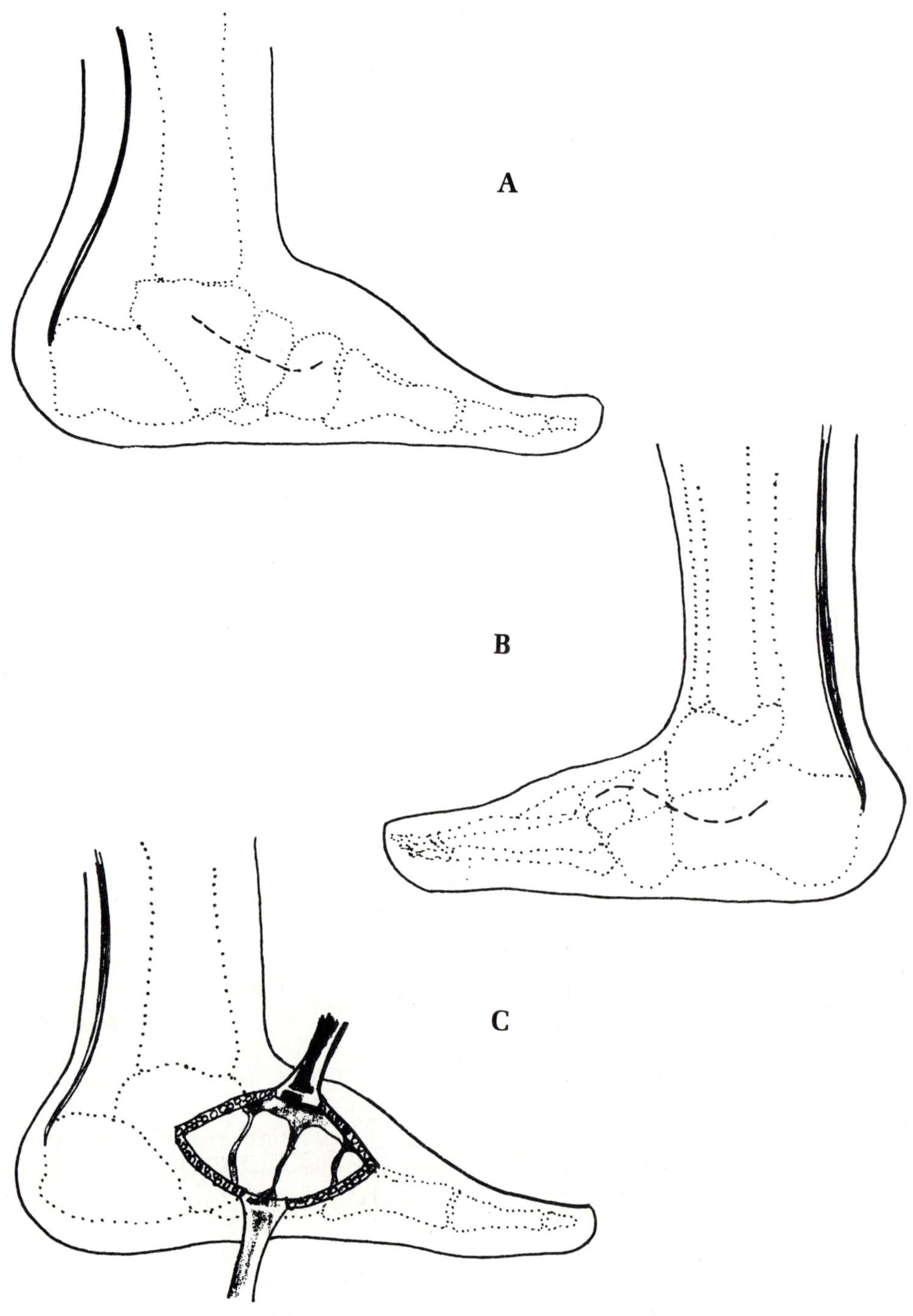

Figure 2. Herndon and Heyman procedure for correction of vertical talus. (A) Broken line indicates skin incision on medial aspect of the foot. (B) Broken line indicates skin incision on lateral aspect of the foot. (C,D) Cap-

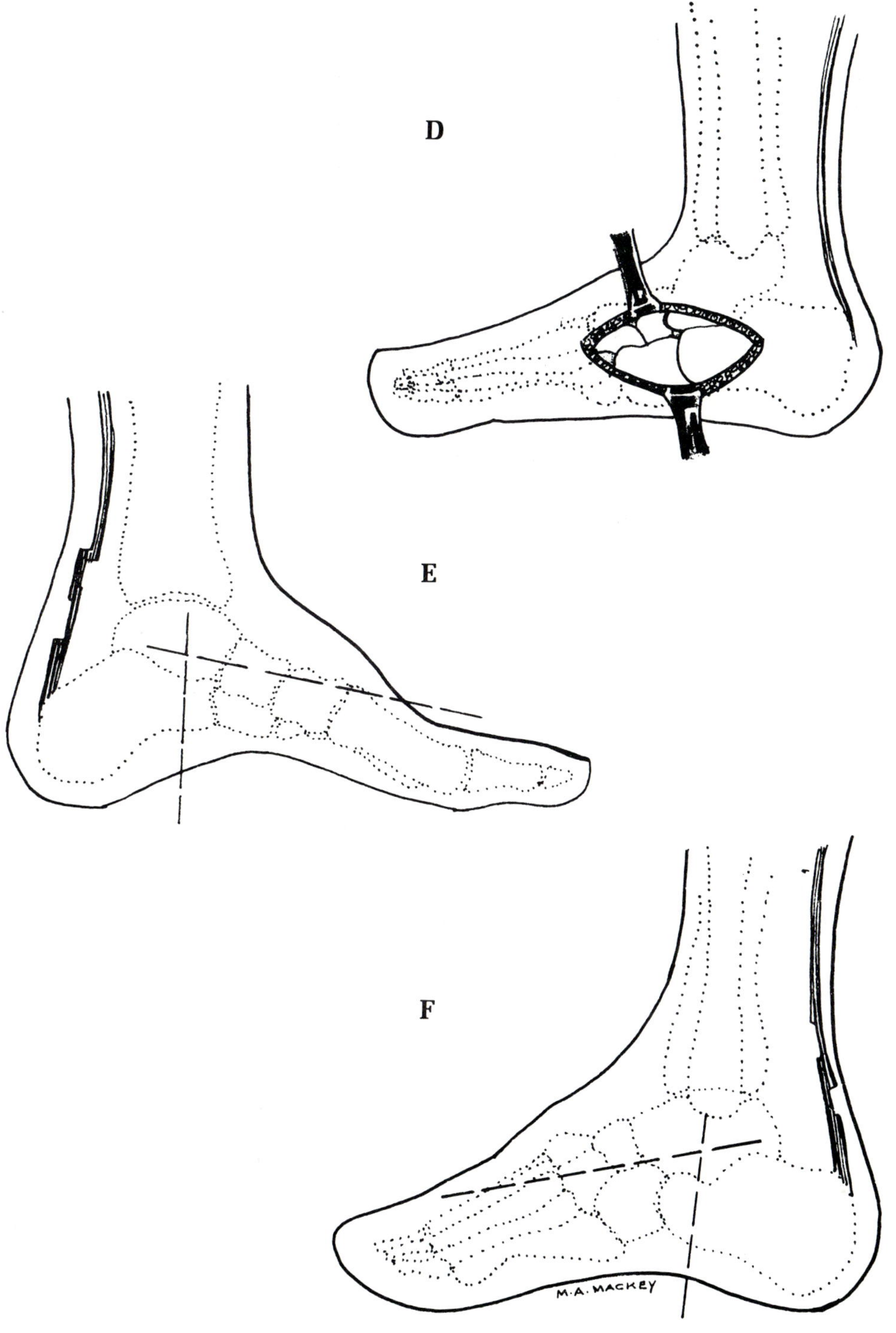

sulotomies of the subtalar and talonavicular joints performed. (E,F) Tendo Achillis lengthened, deformity reduced and Kirschner wires transfixed maintaining correction.

1. Make a medial curved incision over the talus, the dorsally dislocated navicular, and the first cuneiform.
2. Release the ligaments and capsular attachments of the subtalar and talonavicular joints.
3. Reduce the deformity by levering the head of the talus superiorly and the navicular inferiorly, bringing the forefoot into alignment with the calcaneus and correcting the valgus.
4. If necessary, make an S-shaped lateral incision over the sinus tarsi and lengthen the tendons of the peroneals and long toe extensors.
5. Maintain the reduction by two transfixing Kirschner wires; insert one from the base of the first metatarsal through the navicular and into the body of the talus, and the other through the sole of the foot and the calcaneus and into the body or neck of the talus.
6. Close the incisions in the usual manner and apply a cast.
7. Six weeks later, with the wires still in place, lengthen the tendo Achillis and perform a posterior capsulotomy of the ankle joint.
8. Apply a long leg cast. Four weeks after the second operation, the Kirschner wires will be removed and a walking boot cast applied for four months.

References

1. Mau, C.: Muskelbefunde und ihre Bedeutung beim Angeborenen Klumpfussleiden. *Arch. Orthop. Unfallchir.* **29**:292, 1930.
2. Ingram, A.S.: Pollex varus or the thumb clutched hand. Thesis submitted to the American Orthopaedic Association, Feb., 1957.
3. Hark, F.W.: Rocker foot due to congenital subluxation of the talus, *J. Bone Jt. Surg.*, **32-A**:344, 1950.
4. Herndon, C.H., and Heyman, C.H.: Problems in the recognition and treatment of congenital convex pes valgus. *J. Bone Jt. Surg.*, **45-A**:113, 1963.
5. Crenshaw, A.H. (Ed): *Campbell's Operative Orthopaedics*, Vol. 2, C.V. Mosby, St. Louis, 1971, pp. 1922–1927.

Selected Bibliography

Giannestras, N.J.: The congenital rigid flatfoot — Its recognition and treatment in infants. *Orthop. Clinic of N.A.* **4**:49–66, 1973.

Giannestras, N.J.: *Foot Disorders*, Lea & Febiger, Philadelphia, 1973, pp. 286–288.

Osmond-Clarke, H.: Congenital vertical talus. *J. Bone Jt. Surg.*, **38-B**:334, 1956.

Tachdjian, M.O.: *Pediatric Orthopaedics*, Vol. 2, W.B. Saunders, Philadelphia, 1972, pp. 1359–1372.

Weinstein, F.: *Principles and Practice of Podiatry*, Lea & Febiger, Philadelphia, 1968, pp. 214–218.

CHAPTER 14

Arthrodesis of the Ankle

When arthrodesis of the ankle is to be performed, several mechanical factors must be dealt with. A major consideration is the effect of ankle fusion on gait. In most cases, fusion with the foot in the neutral position provides better function than fusion with the foot in equinus. Too great a degree of equinus will cause a halting gait and shortened steps; during walking the affected foot will be pushed forward and the opposing foot will be drawn up from the rear. At the other extreme, a foot in calcaneus after ankle arthrodesis will give a stiffened gait because of the effect of push-off on the calcaneus. Assuming normal muscle strength and joint mobility in the foot, the neutral position provides the best function with walking after ankle fusion. This is so because midtarsal motion will permit forefoot flexion and a more elastic gait.

When arthrodesis of the ankle becomes necessary because of a nontuberculous lesion or a lesion that does not involve the subtalar joint, it is advisable to fuse the talus to the tibia alone, leaving the subtalar joint free. In taking this approach a greater degree of foot mobility is preserved.

Another consideration in performing an ankle arthrodesis is the principle of compression. With the Charnley compression technique, for example, equinus and medial and lateral angulation defects can be corrected.[1] Compression is particularly useful in cases of ankle fracture where bones are poorly or incorrectly reunited. In children, the compression technique is preferred because it accomplishes fusion without damaging the distal tibial epiphyseal plate. Another technique, that developed by Chiunard and Peterson, also involves the principle of compression, but it includes distraction compression of a distal bone graft placed between the talus and the tibia.[2] Like the Charnley technique, this procedure preserves the distal tibial epiphyseal plate, which is a specific advantage to patients in the growth stage.

Additional procedures for ankle arthrodesis include anterior fusion of the tibial talar joint and posterior arthrodesis of the ankle. The latter approach has certain advantages over the former; (1) it has a less traumatic effect on bone and tissue, so posterior ankylosis secondary to tuberculosis will be minimal, and (2) it provides easy access to the tendo Achillis, which may require lengthening if talipes equinus is to be completely corrected.

The final technique presented here is pantalar arthrodesis, which is the treatment of choice when the talus is displaced in the ankle mortise and when flail foot from anterior poliomyelitis must be repaired. The technique combines ankle arthrodesis and triple arthrodesis of the foot.

Charnley Compression Arthrodesis

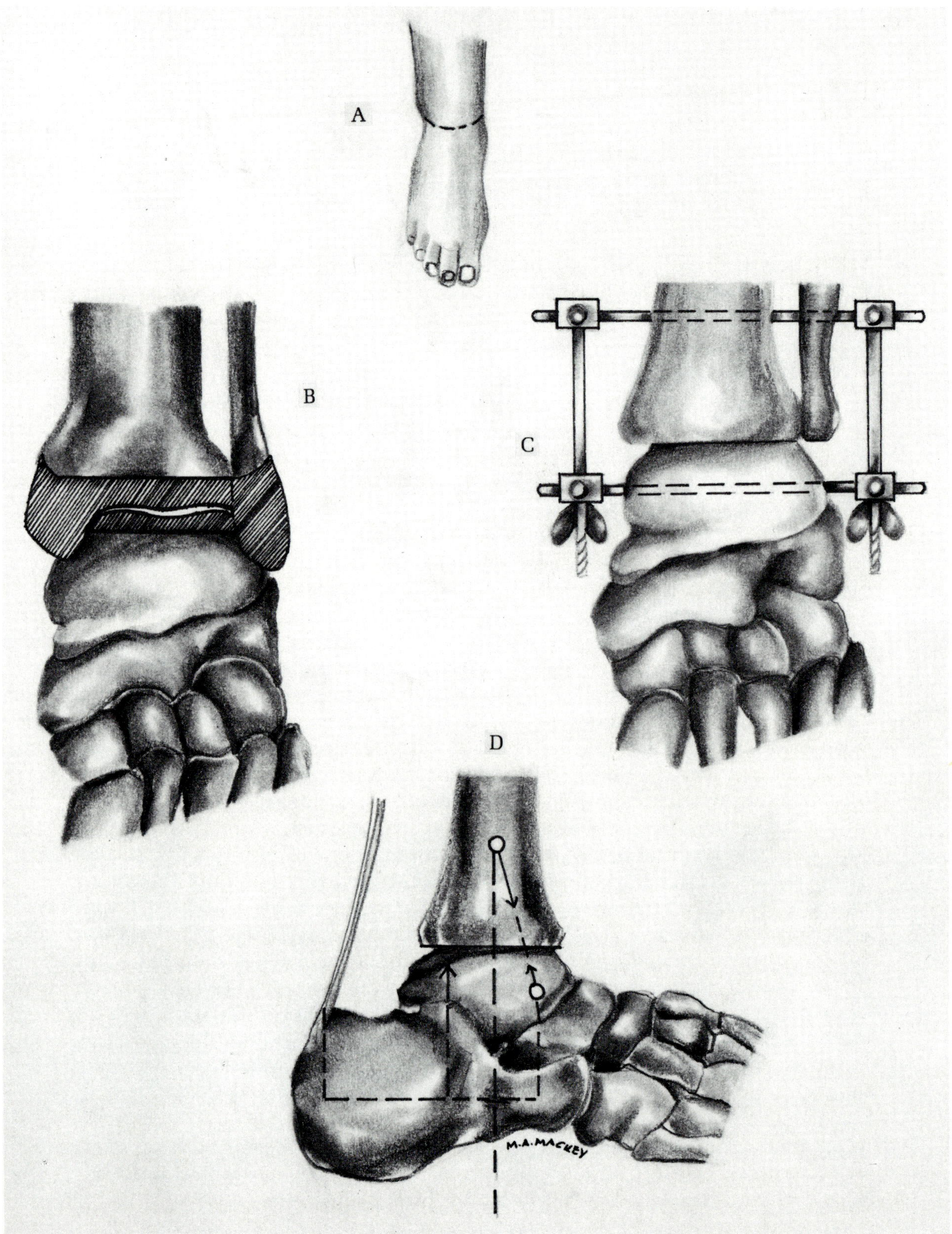

1. Make an incision across the anterior aspect of the ankle joint, extending from 1 cm proximal to the tip of the malleolus to the same position on the other side. The incision is curved distally at its midpoint so that the line of resection of the tendons will not be directly beneath the skin incision.
2. Dissect the skin and subcutaneous tissue proximally to form a thick flap, and expose the extensor tendons.
3. Between thread sutures, divide the tendons of the tibialis anterior, the extensor hallucis longus, the peroneus tertius, and the extensor digitorum communis. Treat the extensor communis as a unit, but take care not to include the distal portion of the peroneus tertius tendon.
4. Cut and tie the anterior tibial vessels, section the nerve, and incise the joint capsule transversely.
5. Expose the distal tibia and the posterior surfaces of the malleoli subperiosteally, and place a periosteal elevator posterior to each malleolus to retract the skin edges.
6. Divide the tibial and fibular collateral ligaments and plantar flex the foot.
7. With a saw, cut the distal ends of the tibia and fibula horizontally. Crack the posterior cortex of the tibia and complete the bone division with an osteotome.
8. Place the foot in the desired position and remove a section of bone approximately ¼ inch thick from the superior surface of the talus.
9. Pass a Steinmann pin through the talus well anterior to the axis of the bone and continue it through the open wound.
   a. The distal pin should be inserted anterior to the transverse axis of the body of the talus to counteract the pull of the tendo Achillis. Be sure not to pierce the subtalar joint with this pin. If the pin is inserted through or posterior to the axis, the force of the tendo Achillis will separate the osseous surfaces anteriorly.
   b. The talus should be displaced as far posteriorly as possible to preserve the prominence of the heel.
   c. After applying the compression clamps to the distal pins to serve as a guide, insert the proximal pin through the shaft of the tibia.
   d. As the clamps are tightened, correct any rotary deformity.
11. Tie the sutures in the tendons and close the skin in the usual manner.
12. Apply a heavily padded plaster cast from the knee to the toes.
13. *After care*. After four to six weeks, the cast, pins, and sutures are removed. A walking boot is worn for an additional four weeks. After eight to ten weeks, the fusion may be sufficiently solid that the patient may wear a shoe without any additional support.

Figure 1 (facing page). Charnley compression arthrodesis of the ankle. (A) Broken line indicates skin incision. (B) Shaded portion indicates bone removed. (C) Arthrodesis of ankle complete with Charnley clamps in place for compression. (D) Distal pin is inserted anterior to the transverse axis of the body of the talus to counteract pull of the tendo Achillis with talus displaced posteriorly to preserve prominence of heel.

Chiunard and Peterson Arthrodesis

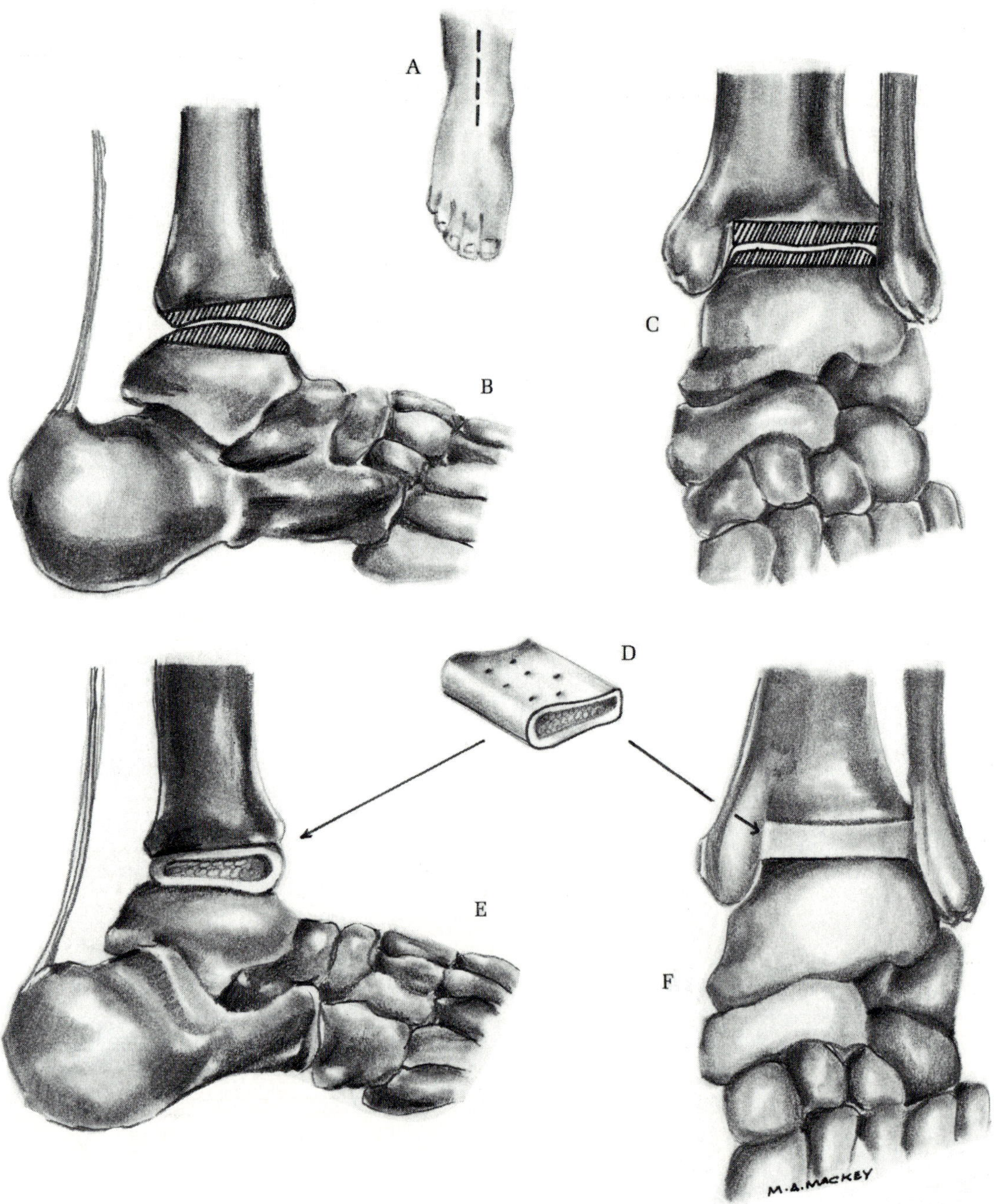

Figure 2. Chuinard and Peterson technique of arthrodesis of the ankle. (A) Broken line indicates skin incision. (B) Shaded area indicates portion of bone and articular surfaces removed (lateral view). (C) Shaded area indicates portion of bone and articular surfaces removed (anterior view). (D) Shaped perforated iliac graft. (E,F) Lateral and anterior views of the ankle with iliac graft in place.

1. Make an anterior longitudinal incision over the joint between the tendons of the extensor longus hallucis and the extensor longus digitorum.
2. Retract the anterior tibial vessels and nerve, and detach the capsule of the ankle joint from the anterior margin of the tibia.
3. With an osteotome and mallet, remove the articular cartilage from the horizontal surfaces of the tibia and talus, but not from the vertical surfaces of these bones or the fibula. Correct any deformity by removing appropriate wedges of bone.
4. With an osteotome the same width as the ankle mortise remove a full thickness graft from the anterior iliac crest as wide as the mortise and as long as the anteroposterior dimension of the ankle. *Do not* include the anterosuperior iliac spine.
5. Tailor the graft to fit the mortise and perforate it with a drill.
6. Manually distract the ankle joint and pound the graft into place with the round rim facing anteriorly and the surfaces of the graft firmly apposed to the surfaces of the tibia and talus.
7. Close the wound in the usual manner.
8. Apply a cast from the base of the toes to the proximal thigh with the knee flexed fifteen degrees.
9. *After care.* After three weeks the cast is either windowed or changed, and the sutures are removed. After six weeks a cast is applied from the base of the toes to below the knee. After two to three months, walking in a cast is started. After three to four months, a short leg brace with a rigid ankle joint is fitted and worn until a solid fusion can be demonstrated roentgenographically.

Anterior Arthrodesis of the Ankle[3]

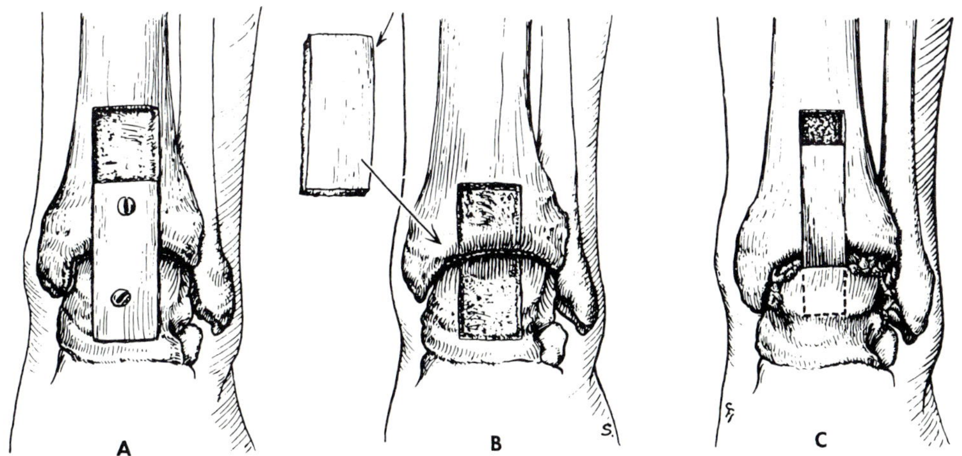

Figure 3. Anterior fusion of ankle. (A) Sliding graft fixed with metal screws. (B) Graft of same dimensions as prepared bed removed from proximal tibia. (C) Sliding graft inserted in cleft in talus; accessory chips in place. (Reproduced with permission from Crenshaw, A.H. (Ed.): *Campbell's Operative Orthopaedics,* Vol. 2, C.V. Mosby, St. Louis, 1971, p. 1126.)

1. Make an anterior incision between the tibialis anticus and the extensors of the toes 3 inches above the ankle down over the dorsum of the foot (Kocher's incision). This incision is simple, direct, and sufficient to expose enough of the ankle joint to produce a solid fusion.
2. The head and neck of the talus are exposed by subperiosteal stripping.
3. The foot is forced into extreme plantar flexion, exposing as much as possible the articular surface of the body of the talus and at least two-thirds of the articular surface of the lower end of the tibia.
4. With a chisel, cut away the entire articular cartilage of the talus, tibia, and fibula exposing enough bone to permit an unobstructed view of the ankle joint.
5. Extreme equinus deformity should be corrected through a separate incision by lengthening the tendo Achillis and performing a posterior capsulotomy. This is rarely necessary, since satisfactory correction of moderate equinus is usually possible after resection of the articular surfaces.
6. Correct any medial or lateral deviation of the talus on the tibia by removing a larger portion of bone from the medial or lateral aspect of the talus or tibia.
7. This intra-articular arthrodesis should be supplemented by one of the following grafts.

   A. *Transplanted Inlay Graft*

   A cortical graft from another part of the tibia is removed and implanted in a window of equal dimensions that has been cut in the anterior aspect of the tibia and talus. It should be so placed as to block dorsiflexion at the proper angle for walking. To obtain early and more certain fusion and to prevent displacement of the graft, insert metal screws through the graft into the talus and tibia. Fill any dead space between the malleoli and the body of the talus with cancellous or cortical chip grafts.

   B. *Sliding Inlay Graft (Preferred)*

   Remove a full thickness cortical graft, 1 inch wide and 2 inches long, from the tibia immediately proximal to the joint surface. Cut a gutter of suitable dimensions in the anterior part of the body and the superior surface of the neck of the talus. Holding the talus and the tibia in proper alignment, move the sliding graft from the tibia distally across the anterior surface of the joint and countersink its distal half into the gutter in the talus. Accessory bone chips are used to fill any dead space between the malleoli and the body of the talus.

8. Close the wound in the usual manner.
9. Press the denuded articular surfaces of the talus into the mortise of the ankle. To stabilize the joint, Steinmann pins and Charnley clamps are almost always used, as described earlier in Charnley compression arthrodesis.
10. After care also is the same as for the Charnley compression arthrodesis.

Arthrodesis of the Tibial-Talar Joint[4]

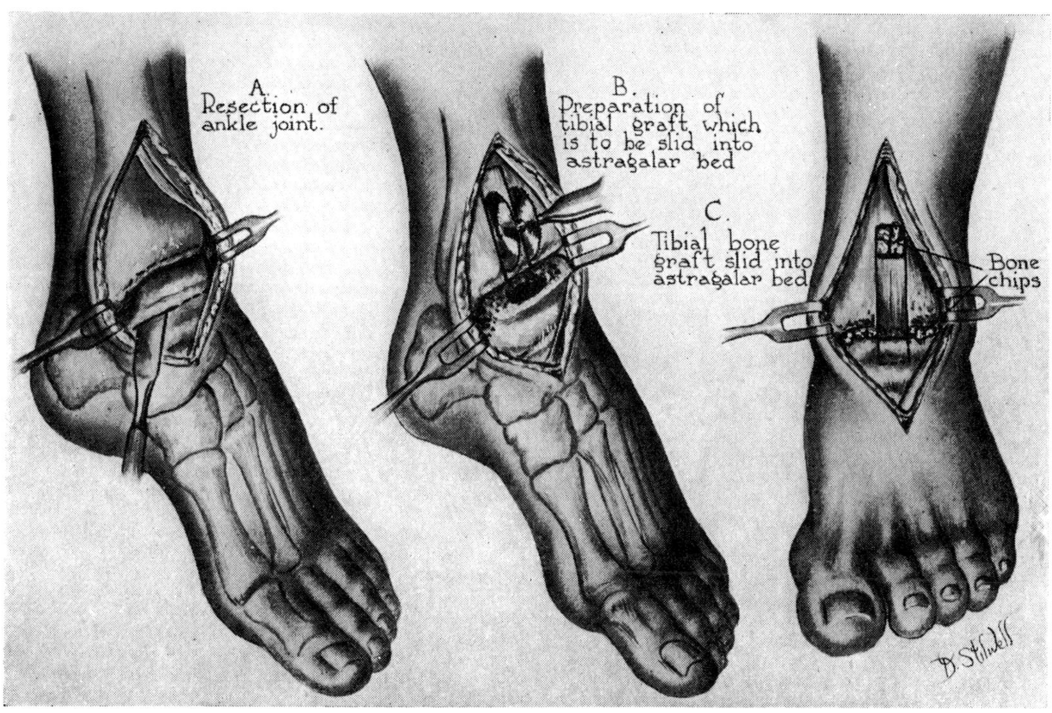

Figure 4. (Reproduced with permission from Steindler, A.: *Orthopedic Operations: Indications, Technique, and End Results,* Charles C Thomas, Springfield, Ill., 1940, p. 327.)

1. An anterior incision is made between the tibialis anticus and the extensors of the toes, 3 inches above the ankle joint and down over the dorsum of the foot (Kocher's incision).
2. The head and neck of the talus are exposed by periosteal stripping.
3. The foot is forced into extreme plantar flexion, exposing as much as possible of the articular surface of the body of the talus, and at least two-thirds of the articular surface of the lower end of the tibia.
4. A deep groove is made into the anterior surface of the tibia to receive the graft taken from the tibia. This groove is continued over the body into the neck of the talus, one-quarter to one-third of an inch deep and just wide enough to receive a good tibial graft.
5. The tibial bone graft is slid into the talar bed.
6. Fill any dead space between the malleoli and the body of the talus with cancellous or cortical chip grafts.
7. Close the wound in the usual manner.
8. Steinmann pins and Charnley clamps are almost always used for compression and stabilization.
9. After care is the same as for Charnley compression arthrodesis.

Posterior Arthrodesis of the Ankle[3]

I. Extra-articular Type

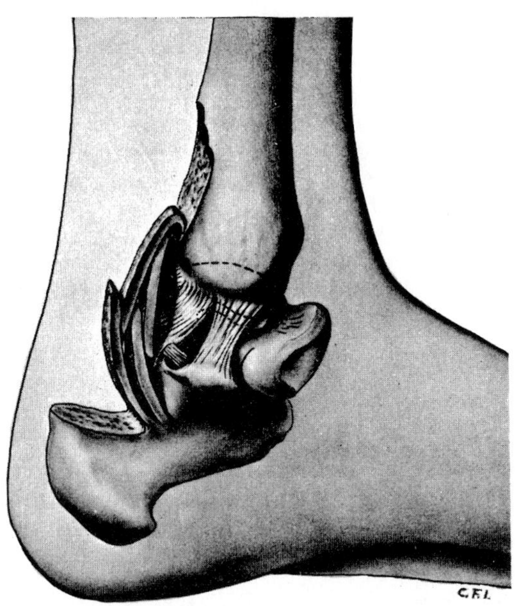

Figure 5. (Reproduced with permission from Crenshaw, A.H. (Ed.): *Campbell's Operative Orthopaedics*, Vol. 2, C.V. Mosby, St. Louis, 1971, p. 1132.)

1. An incision is made 3 inches long over the posterior aspect of the ankle joint medial and parallel with the tendo Achillis.
2. The incision is carried down between the tendo Achillis and the posterior ankle capsule.
3. The flexor longus hallucis is retracted medially. *Do not* incise the posterior ankle capsule.
4. With an osteotome, turn large flaps of bone distally from the posterior aspect of the tibia and proximally from the superior surface of the calcaneus, overlapping them successively at the level of the ankle joint to provide a massive extra-articular bridge across the joint.
5. The incision is closed in the usual manner.
6. The foot is immobilized in a plaster cast from the toes to well above the knee, with the foot at a right angle to the leg. To allow for swelling, a window is cut in the cast over the dorsum of the foot, then is replaced and held loosely with bandages.
7. *After care.* Four weeks after operation another snug-fitting boot cast is applied; or if the reaction has been mild, a walking cast will suffice. Weight-bearing is cautiously resumed. Full weight-bearing is usually de-

layed for eight to twelve weeks after surgery. Cast immobilization is continued until both the ankle and the subtalar joints are solidly arthrodesed.

According to Campbell, results are excellent. The patient generally acquires an almost normal gait, although walking on irregular surfaces may be difficult.

II. Intra-articular Type (used only when the subtalar and ankle joints are both involved).

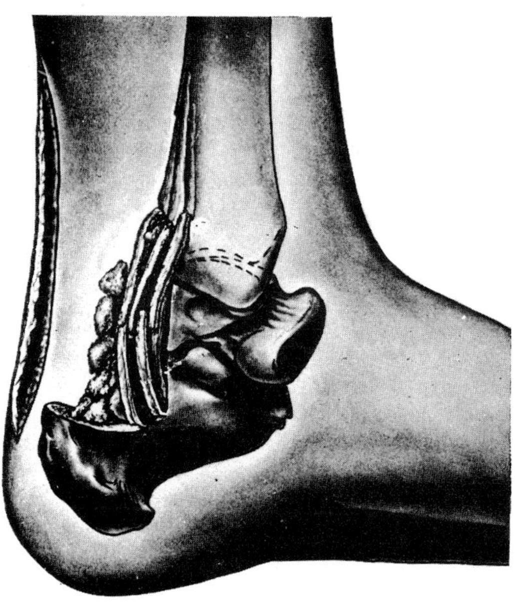

Figure 6. (Reproduced with permission from Crenshaw, A.H. (Ed.) *Campbell's Operative Orthopaedics*, Vol. 2, C.V. Mosby, St. Louis, 1971, p. 1134.)

1. Incision and exposure are the same as for the extra-articular type.
2. The capsule is incised transversely, and the posterior extremity of the talus and the articular surfaces of the posterior aspect of the ankle joint are removed.
3. The surfaces of the subtalar joint are denuded if it is involved.
4. Bone flaps are then turned distally from the tibia and proximally from the calcaneus, but are impacted so as to come in contact not only with each other but also with the posterior surface of the talus.
5. Incision closed in the usual manner.
6. Casting and after care are the same as for the extra-articular type.

Pantalar Arthrodesis[4]

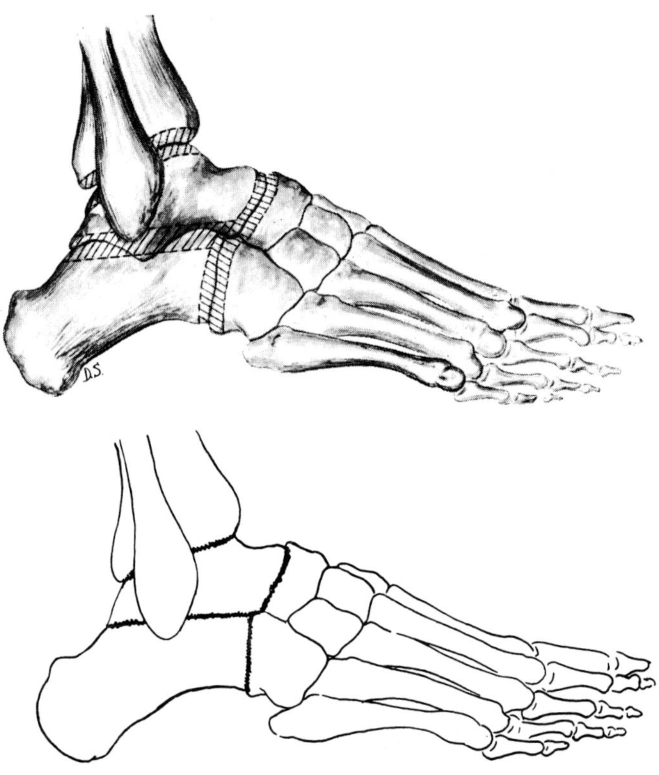

Figure 7. (Reproduced with permission from Steindler, A.: *Orthopedic Operations: Indications, Technique, and End Results,* Charles C Thomas, Springfield, Ill., 1940, p. 330.)

1. An anterolateral incision is made just anterior to the tip of the lateral malleolus. This incision is preferred to the Kocher incision because it does not disturb the inferior ligaments of the talus any more than is necessary and it does not interfere with the blood supply to the talus.
2. Retract the extensors medially and divide the lateral ligaments of the ankle. Open the ankle joint by extreme supination and abduction of the foot, as in the Whitman talectomy (see Chapter 7).
3. The subtalar joint and the ankle joint are exposed.
4. The talus is mobilized by dividing all ligaments to the neighboring bone except the inferior ligament.
5. The articular cartilage of the tibia, the fibula, and the body of the talus is removed.
6. Pull the talus proximally and remove the cartilage from the subtalar joint, including the facet of the sustentaculum tali.
7. Denude the talonavicular and calcaneocuboid joints.
8. Correct any lateral deformity by removing the bone from the subtalar and midtarsal joints.
9. Be sure that all the bone surfaces fit together well and that the foot is in satisfactory position.

10. Incision is closed in the usual manner.
11. Casting and after care are the same as for triple arthrodesis.

References

1. Charnley, J.: Compression arthrodesis of the ankle and shoulder. *J. Bone Surg.*, **33-B**:180, 1951.
2. Chuinard, E.G., and Peterson, R.E.: Distraction-compression bone graft arthrodesis of the ankle. A method applicable to children. *J. Bone Jt. Surg.*, **45-A**:481, 1963.
3. Crenshaw, A.H. (Ed.): *Campbell's Operative Orthopaedics*, C.V. Mosby, St. Louis, 1971, pp. 1125–1134.
4. Steindler, A.: *Orthopedic Operations*, Charles C Thomas, Springfield, Ill., 1940, pp. 327–330.

Selected Bibliography

Campbell, W.C.: An operation for the induction of osseous fusion of the ankle joint. *Am. J. Surg.*, **6:**588, 1929.

Campbell, W.C.: Fusion of tuberculous joints. Surg. *Clin. North Am.*, **10**:823, 1930.

Goldstein, L.A., and Dickerson, R.C.: *Atlas of Orthopaedic Surgery*, Vol. 2, C.V. Mosby, St. Louis, 1974, pp. 882–886.

CHAPTER 15

Total Ankle Replacement Arthroplasties

Total ankle replacement has the combined advantages of relieving pain associated with ankle arthrodesis and restoring joint mobility. Although it is a fairly new technique, and there is no established criterion for age, it has been performed with success in patients with advanced arthritis.

The four procedures detailed here differ according to the design of the prosthesis employed. Most devices have a talar component, made of stainless steel or of a chrome-cobalt-molybdenum alloy, and a tibial component, constructed of high-density polyethylene.[1] Implants are fixed with methyl methacrylate.

Indications for total ankle replacement include traumatic rheumatoid arthritis, osteoarthritis, and failure of such procedures as subtalar arthrodesis. In the presence of localized infection (past or present), neuropathy, ligament instability, or vascular impairment, total ankle replacement is contraindicated.

There are several major concerns that the foot surgeon must consider when contemplating the introduction of a foreign prosthetic component. Of utmost importance is that the surgery successfully restore adequate ankle joint motion to permit a normal gait cycle. Such motion must consist of a minimum of 10 degrees of dorsiflexion and 20 degrees of plantar flexion. Thus, approximately 30 degrees of sagittal plane motion is necessary at the ankle when the subtalar joint is in a neutral position to allow normal locomotion. This degree of dorsiflexor motion is required at the ankle when the knee extends just before the heel is lifted from the ground. It is this dorsiflexor motion which allows the tibia to move 10 degrees forward from vertical without creating a premature heel left or a pronated foot. Secondly, the surgeon must look beyond the arthritic joint and be fully aware that the coexisting deformities of varus, valgus equinus and calcaneus will inevitably lead to a poor result if neglected. The surgeon must also evaluate the type of arthritis and be wary of systemic manifestations that may doom the surgery to failure. Thirdly, the surgeon must make every effort to achieve a surgery which creates stability. Such stability may well rest in the design of the prosthetic component itself. One must utilize an implant design which affords intrinsic stability against both medial and lateral forces and thus prohibits extreme loading, wearing and loosening of the prosthesis. The prosthetics which utilize intramedullary pinning or screws should be avoided. A common problem of stability can be easily avoided if the surgeon preoperatively evaluates the existing ligamentous support of the ankle. A prosthetic should never be contemplated if the ankle is without ligamentous support. Lastly, the surgeon must make every effort to salvage as much bone as possible when performing the procedure, so that if arthrodesis becomes necessary it can be performed inconsequentially.

Scholz Technique—Angular Total Ankle Prosthesis[2,3]

Talar component, cobalt chromium alloy; tibial component, ultra-high molecular weight polyethylene.

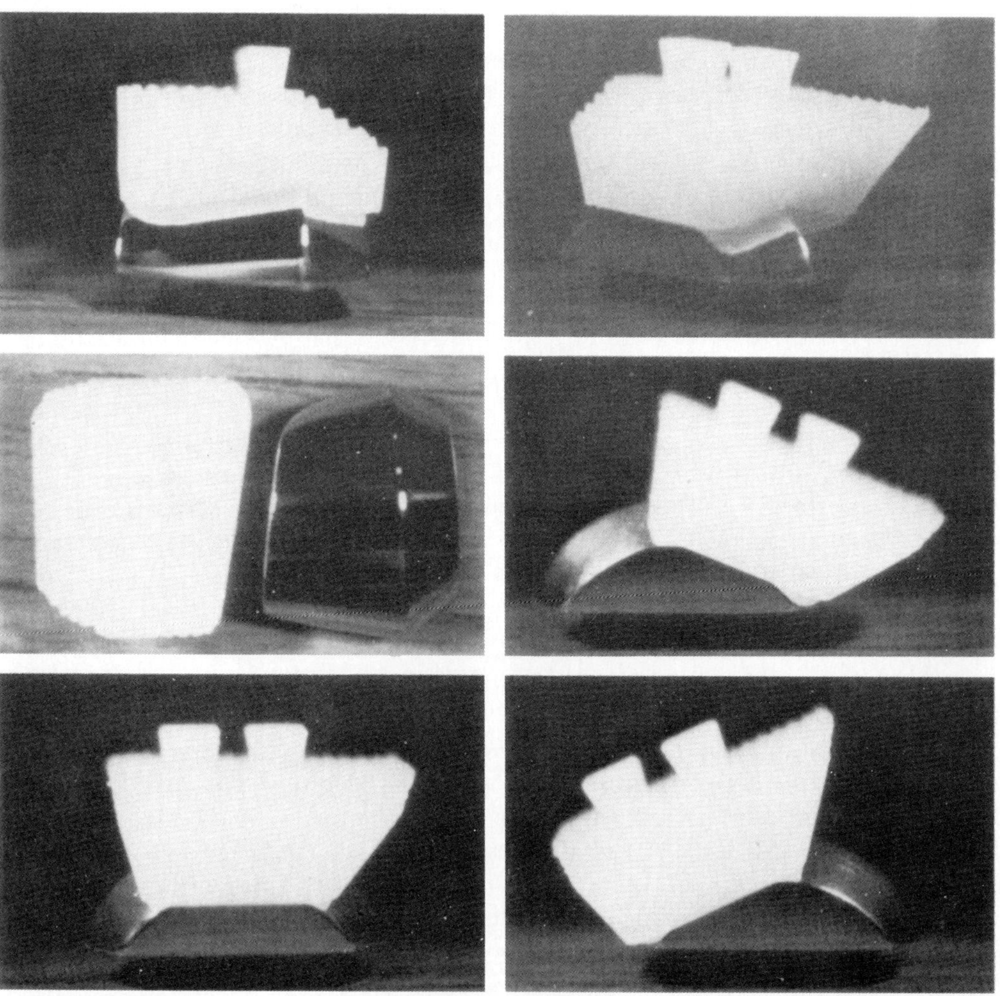

Figure 1. The angular total contact ankle prosthesis. (Reproduced with permission from Bateman, J.E. (Ed.): *Foot Science*, W.B. Saunders, Philadelphia, 1976, p. 109.)

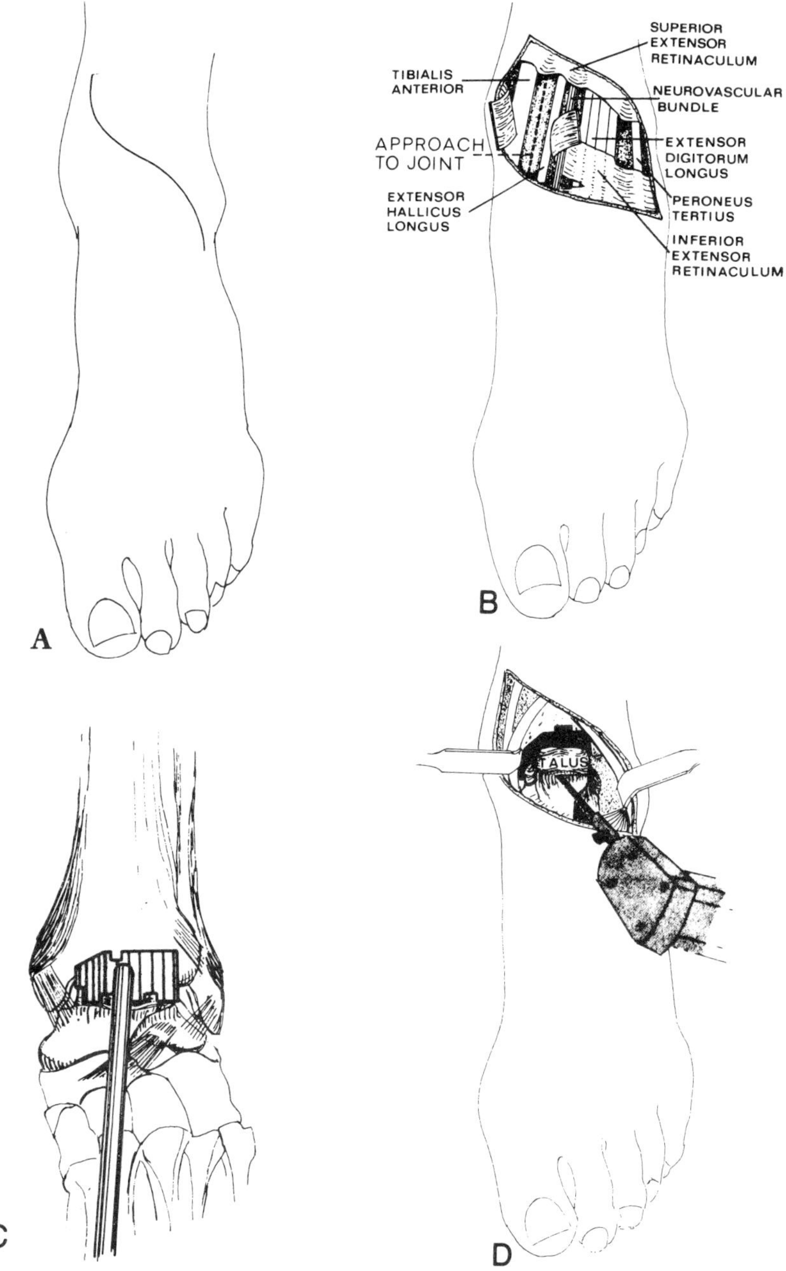

Figure 2. (A) The ankle is exposed through an anterior "lazy-S" incision. (B) The interval developed into the joint is between the anterior tibial and extensor hallucis longus tendons. (C) A trial block gauge helps determine the amount of bone and configuration of the osteotomies. It should fit snugly into the resected surfaces and the long lever arm should project between the first and second metatarsals. This compensates for tibial torsion and helps project the articular components to the line of progression of the body. (D) A reciprocating saw removes the desired portion and configuration of respective surfaces of the tibia and dome of talus. (Reproduced with permission from Bateman, J.E. (Ed.): *Foot Science*, W.B. Saunders, Philadelphia, 1976, pp. 118-119.) *Continued on next page.*

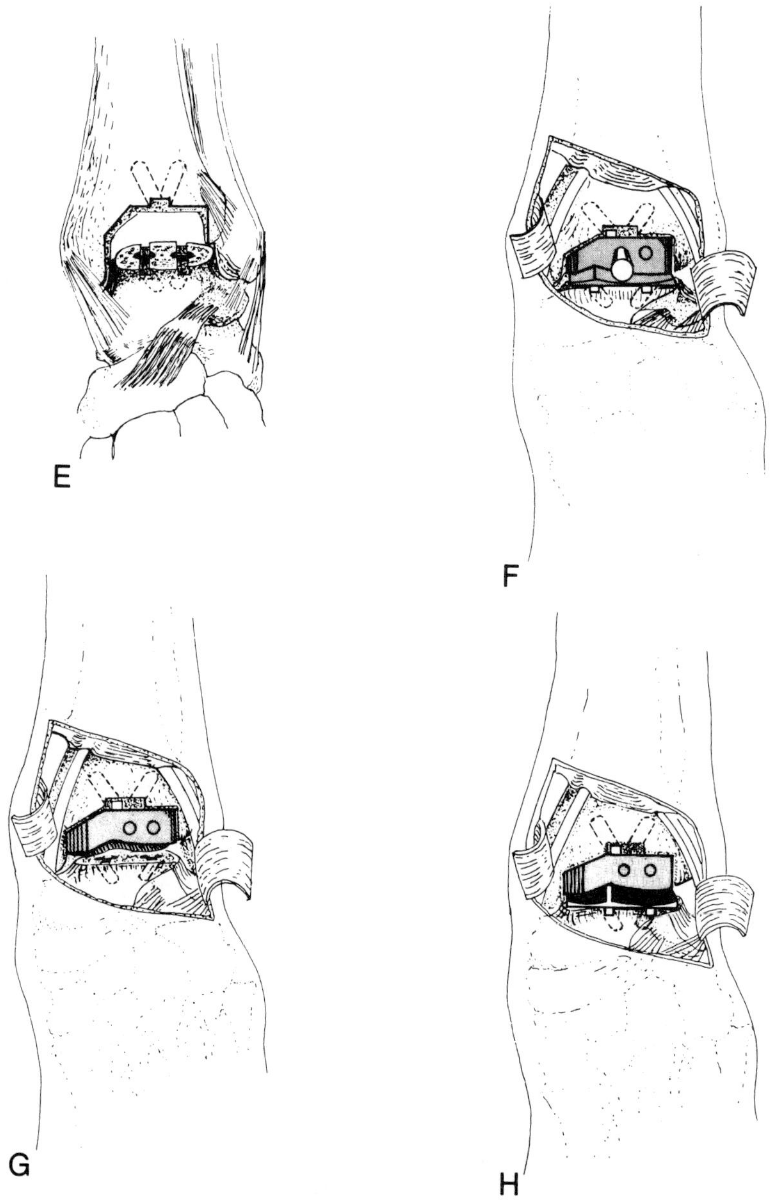

Figure 2 (continued). (E) The configuration of the resected tibial and talar surfaces. A single slot is cut into the tibia and two into the talus. Holes are projected into the surfaces for added purchase of methacrylate. The trial gauge block should fit snugly into this space. (F) The trial components are inserted to check alignment and motion. The removable lever arm should project toward an interval between the great and second toes. (G) The tibial component is cemented initially. The removable lever arm can also be utilized to position the prosthesis. The trial talar component may be slipped beneath the cemented tibial component to maintain pressure while the cement hardens with the foot in a neutral to slight dorsiflexed position and then removed. (H) The talar component is then cemented into place. (Reproduced with permission from Bateman, J.E. (Ed.): *Foot Science,* W.B. Saunders, Philadelphia, 1976, pp. 118–119.)

1. Anterior exposure of the ankle via a "lazy S" curvilinear incision.
2. Begin incision on the anteromedial aspect of the ankle, curve it obliquely across the tibiotalar joint and distally along the anterolateral aspect of the dorsum of the foot.
3. Continue down to the periosteum of the tibia and, with the use of a reciprocating saw, remove a rectangular portion of the tibia perpendicular to its long axis.
4. Next place foot in neutral position, and resect a portion of the talar dome parallel to the tibial surface.
5. If foot is in equinus a posterior capsulotomy can be performed. A TAL is usually deferred for early ambulation.
6. Trial gauge block is inserted to determine if the space is adequate and to check alignment. It should fit snugly into the prepared cavity, and the lever arm should project between the first and second metatarsals.
7. Marked slots in the template are used to remove one rectangular osteotomy slot from the tibia and two from the talus, to accommodate the non-articulating projections of the components.
8. The trial prosthesis is then inserted and observed for snug articulation. Radiographs may be helpful at this time.
9. Holes are also drilled into both tibial and talus to insure methacrylate hold.
10. The tibial component is inserted, positioned and excessive soft cement removed. It is advantageous to place the talar component (without cement) as this helps maintain the desired position of the tibial component.
11. Talar component is then removed, tibial component is checked for stability, and the process repeated while positioning the talar component.
12. Ankle checked for stability and motion. Radiographs taken.
13. Wound closed in layers and closed suction drains inserted. A short leg cast is applied with foot in neutral position.

TPR Total Ankle Replacement[4]

Talar component, stainless steel or cobalt chromium alloy; tibial component, ultra-high molecular weight polyethylene.

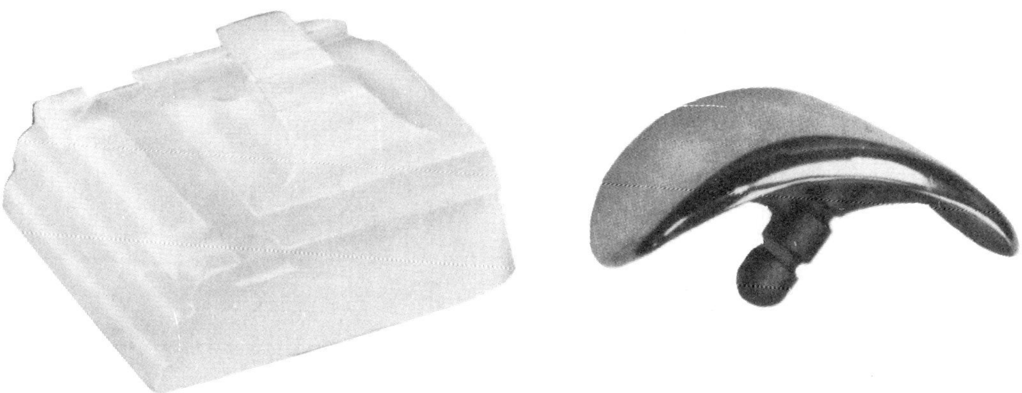

Figure 3. (Reproduced with permission of Richards Manufacturing Company, Inc., Memphis, TN.)

1. Anterior incision is made parallel and slightly lateral to the extensor hallucis longus. The incision, 10–12 cm in length, runs longitudinally along the distal one-third of the leg, across the ankle joint, and extends to the talonavicular joint.
2. The superficial branch of the peroneal nerve is identified along with the dorsalis pedis artery. The peroneal nerve, the anterior tibial tendon, the extensor hallucis longus tendon, and the dorsalis pedis artery are retracted medially. The common extensor tendon and the remaining soft tissues are retracted to the lateral aspect of the wound after the transverse fascia has been sectioned longitudinally.
3. The dissection is then carried down to the periosteum on the anterior cortex of the tibia. All soft tissue (including the joint capsule) is then dissected, subperiosteally, down across the ankle joint and out to the talonavicular joint.
4. The lateral branch of the dorsalis pedis is sectioned.
5. A small V-shaped section of the anterior tibial is excised to obtain better exposure of the joint.
6. Cervical laminar spreaders are then inserted, the joint inspected, and a 1 cm section of the dome of the talus is removed.
7. Various sizes of the Spacer-Template are then inserted into the ankle mortise to determine the width and thickness of the trial prosthesis.
8. The subchondral bone of the distal tibia is then excised with an air burr for a depth of approximately 1–1¼ cm.
9. The horizontal arm of the Spacer-Template should make a 90 degree angle with the anterior cortex of the tibia. If the angle is less than 90 degrees, additional bone should be removed from the posterior aspect of the tibial to preserve the normal axis of motion in dorsiflexion and plantar flexion. The vertical arm is positioned to parallel the anterior cortex of the tibia so that the Spacer-Template will not be in either varus or valgus.
10. A 3/16 inch drill hole is made through the Spacer-Template into the distal tibia. A notch is placed in the exact center of the anterior tibial cortex. The notch is enlarged to accommodate the post of the Tibial Component.
11. The posterior aspect of the tibial prosthesis is curved to allow easier insertion. The tibial implant has skirts on the medial and lateral aspect to prevent metal contact against the medial or lateral malleolus. The implant is surrounded by the medial, lateral and posterior tibial cortex.
12. The Talus Template is then driven into place after all spurring along the junction of the body and the neck of the talus has been removed. The center of the Talus Template is aligned with the notch in the anterior cortex of the tibia. Through the hole in the template, a ¼ inch hole is drilled into the body of the talus to a depth of 1½–2 cm.
13. The slots in the Talus Marking Template are marked with methylene blue.
14. An air burr is then used for deepening and widening the recess in the talus for accepting the post and gusset of the Trial Talus Implant. The recess should be enlarged to allow sufficient space for insertion of the implant and an adequate amount of methylmethacrylate for firm fixation.
15. The Trial Talus Implant is then inserted to ensure proper seating and alignment.
16. The wound is irrigated with antibiotic solution and cleaned of all bone

debris. The tourniquet is then inflated, all bleeding controlled and preparation for the final implant is begun. At this time the methylmethacrylate is prepared.

17. The final Tibial Component is inserted first and excess cement is removed. The final Talus Component is then inserted. All excess cement from the posterior joint should be removed. All impaction should be done utilizing a driver with a plastic head.
18. Before the cement hardens, to ensure proper alignment of the implants, pressure is applied to the plantar surface of the foot with ankle in a neutral position. Pressure is maintained until the cement hardens.
19. Final implant positioning is then checked with "range of motion" test.
20. The periosteum and joint capsule is closed; closed suction drainage is used, all bleeding controlled, and the wound is closed in the usual manner.

Smith Total Ankle Replacement[5]

Talar component, polyethylene; tibial component, stainless steel.

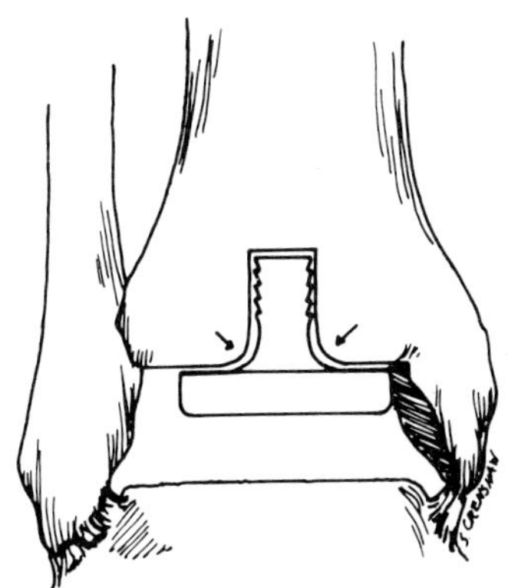

Figure 4. Tibial component. (Reproduced with permission of Wright Manufacturing Company, Arlington, TN, and Richard C. Smith, M.D., San Pedro, CA.)

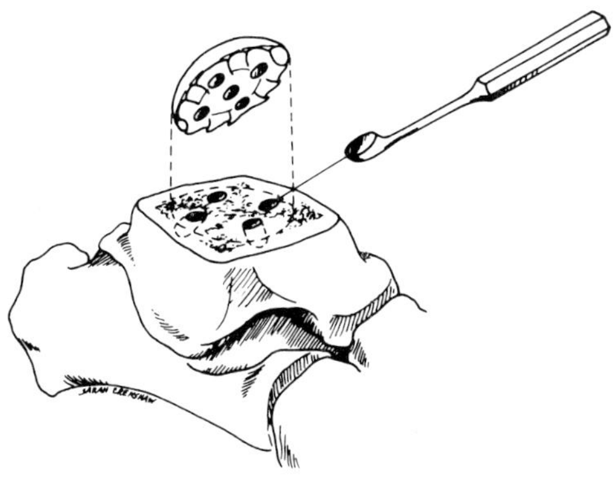

Figure 5. Talar component. (Reproduced with permission of Wright Manufacturing Company, Arlington, TN, and Richard C. Smith, M.D., San Pedro, CA.)

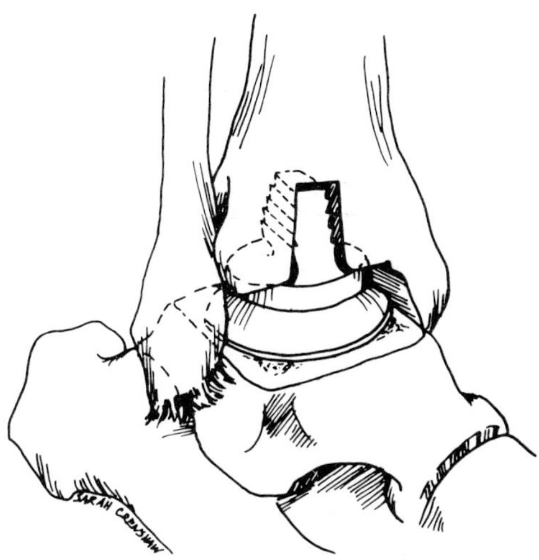

Figure 6. Total ankle. (Reproduced with permission of Wright Manufacturing Company, Arlington, TN, and Richard C. Smith, M.D., San Pedro, CA.)

1. An anterolateral approach is made to the tibiotalar joint, with the common toe extensors and the neurovascular bundle being retracted medially. The anterolateral malleolar and lateral tarsal arteries are sacrificed.
2. When the joint space is exposed, along with the dome of the talus, note the location of the anterior talofibular ligament, which is to be preserved.
3. Using the "spool-like" template, the proposed osteotomy sites in the talus and tibia are visualized, with the template held in position proximal to the talofibular ligament.
4. The two coronal osteotomy sites are then marked with an osteotome, and the osteotomies completed with a narrow-bladed oscillating saw of adequate depth. Care should be taken to avoid penetration of the integrity of the posterior medial neurovascular bundle.
5. Place template into the newly formed space. The template confirms the adequacy of the height of the prepared space. In addition, it aids centering the two prosthetic components; its smaller upper diameter equals the diameter of the metal tibial cut prosthesis, and its larger lower diameter equals the diameter of the polyethylene talar dome prosthesis.
6. The template is positioned between the osteotomized tibia and talus so that it is reasonably centered on the A-P and lateral centerline of the tibia, and the opening of the template is faced anteriorly. A section of bone equal in width and depth to the template opening, and 1.5 cm in length, is removed from the distal tibia with the oscillating saw.
7. Deepen the cut sufficiently in the cancellous bone of the tibial posteriorly to accept the posterior half of the tibial prosthesis sagittal fin. Preserve a shelf, or lip of cortical bone, to interlock with the notch opening of the prosthesis.
8. Round off the corners at the junction of the coronal and sagittal cuts in the anterior-posterior view, to allow for proper seating of the tibial prosthesis.

9. At least four obliquely directed radiating curette holes are made on the floor of the osteotomized talus to provide fixation points for methylmethacrylate cement in seating the polyethylene talar prosthesis later.
10. With both trial components temporarily in place, a trial range of motion is attempted. When the range of motion is satisfactory, the trial components are removed and the wound thoroughly irrigated. The tourniquet is released to monitor the integrity of the posterior tibial artery. Bleeding should be controlled if present. The leg is re-elevated and the tourniquet re-inflated.
11. The first batch of cement is prepared. When in a dough-like state, a small portion of cement is worked into the prepared surface of the tibia and the tibial prosthesis pushed into place with the thumb. There should be approximately 3 mm thickness of cement between the bone and the shoulder of the tibial prosthesis when the prosthesis is in place. Any excess cement is carefully removed with a curette. The prosthesis is held firmly in place until the cement sets.
12. The second batch of cement is prepared. A small patty of cement is placed on the talar prosthesis undersurface and pressure applied to force cement into the grooves and holes. The talar prosthesis is then placed on the prepared talar surface and pushed lightly into place. Prevent exuding cement posteriorly. The talar prosthesis should be positioned directly under and in alignment with the tibial prosthesis. A trial range of motion is accomplished gently. The amount of cement between the interface of bone and prosthesis should be no more than 3 mm. Any excess exuded cement should be removed. The ankle should be held in neutral stance while the cement sets.
13. The wound is again irrigated and a medium or large suction type drain is placed into the operative site. A layered closure is carefully done, and a dressing applied. A large, bulky, pressure type dressing with a posterior splint has been utilized with good results in keeping post-op edema to a minimum. The drain is pulled within 24 hours, and the bulky dressing is exchanged for a short leg cast at about the fifth day post-op. Short periods of weight-bearing can begin when tolerated, but elevation should be encouraged as much as possible for at least two weeks to ensure skin healing.

Oregon Total Ankle Replacement[6]

Talar component, Zimaloy (cast cobalt chromium molybdenum alloy); tibial component, ultra-high molecular weight polyethylene.

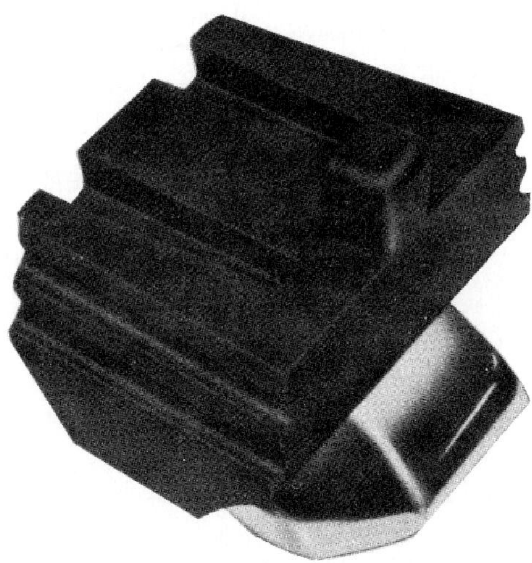

Figure 7 (Reproduced with permission of Zimmer-USA-International, Warsaw, IN.)

1. Using an anterior approach, an incision is made just lateral to the anterior tibial tendon. The incision should extend approximately 4½ inches above and 1½ inches below the ankle joint. Next, the superior and inferior retinacula are cut. Carefully, the external hallucis longus and the vascular bundle are displaced laterally with blunt retraction. The anterior tibial is displaced medially in the same fashion.
2. A long incision is made through the periosteum, the capsule of the ankle joint and onto the talus. Using a curved osteotome, the periosteum and the ankle capsule are stripped medially and laterally.
3. The distal tibia is resected first because of the inherent tightness of the joint. The center of the talus is marked with an osteotome. A corresponding mark is then made on the anterior edge of the distal tibia. The tibial resection guide is then positioned with its central notch over the marked center of the talus. The markings on the prongs of the guide should be at the level of the ankle joint and the long handle be held parallel with the long axis of the tibia. The area inside the prongs of the guide and the notched area are marked with methylene blue. A small reciprocating or osteotomy saw is used for resecting the cortical bone in the marked area. The resection is carried to the posterior cortex in a plane perpendicular to the axis of the tibia.
4. A burr or a small rongeur may be used for bone removal. As the resection is carried posteriorly, it should be noted that the fibula may intrude significantly into the distal tibia. The fibula should not be disturbed. The long axis of the tibia should bisect the axis of flexion (horizontal). If the

tibial prosthesis is placed too anteriorly, the dome of the talar prosthesis would strike the posterior margin of the tibial prosthesis and result in failure. The area marked through the notch of the tibial resection guide is then cut to about ⅜ inch from the anterior lip of the tibia.

5. The foot is aligned and the talar drill guide is placed centrally over the talus with the handle parallel to the bottom of the foot. A 3/16 inch drill with the drill stop in place is used to drill a vertical hole into the superior surface of the talus.
6. The talar resection guide is inserted into the ankle joint. The small peg on the undersurface of the instrument is fitted into the hole in the talus. The handle of the guide should be held in line with the second metatarsal.
7. The exposed medial and lateral borders of the talus are next resected. The planes of these resections should be in the same slope as the sides of the guide. Care should be taken not to carry the resection too distally in order to preserve the ligaments.
8. The cartilage on the superior surface of the talus is removed. When viewed anteriorly, the medial and lateral slopes of the resected talus should be identical and the superior surface of the talus should be flat.
9. To check the resection of the talus, the provisional talar prosthesis is fitted on the talus. The prosthesis should seat firmly on the talus and should not rock when pressure is applied.
10. With the provisional talar prosthesis in place, a tibial spacer of appropriate thickness is inserted into the joint. If the distal tibia is resected properly, the handle of the tibia spacer should be parallel to the anterior ledge of the provisional talar prosthesis. The anterior talar lip of the tibial spacer should rest just above the horizontal groove of the provisional talar prosthesis when the foot is in the neutral position. If the horizontal groove cannot be visualized, the tibial spacer should be removed and a burr used to remove only bony intrusions on the ceiling or posterior corners of the tibial recess. A minimal gap should exist between the superior surface of the tibial spacer and the resected tibia.
11. The tibial spacer is removed and the ankle joint is distracted to receive the provisional tibial prosthesis corresponding to the tibial spacer of choice. The range of motion and the laxity of the joint are tested. The fibula should not contact the provisional tibial prosthesis.
12. Osteophytes, if present, are removed from the medial and lateral malleoli with a small rongeur. Any osteophytes located in the posterior tibia are carefully removed with a curved osteotome and a small rongeur. The main portion of the posterior cortex and the capsule should be left intact.
13. The cement is mixed and a small amount is applied to the talus, taking care to pack cement into the cement holes. A thin layer of cement is then applied to the under-surface of the talar prosthesis and installed.
14. After the talar prosthesis is cemented in place, the ankle joint is carefully distracted and the provisional tibial prosthesis removed. A second batch of cement is mixed and a small amount is inserted into the tibial bed, again carefully packing cement into the holes previously prepared. Cement is applied to the medial and superior surfaces of the tibial prosthesis, packing the respective fixation grooves. *No cement should be applied laterally*. Any cement between the fibula and the prosthesis is susceptible to failure because of fibular movement. Care should be taken

to avoid the presence of cement in this area unless the fibula is fused to the tibia. The joint is again gently distracted and the tibial component is inserted and cemented in place. Again, excess and exposed cement are removed. The foot is held in neutral position until the cement has hardened.

15. The range of motion of the ankle is checked and any source of impingement eliminated. The joint is irrigated to wash out any debris.
16. The incision is closed in layers over small hemovac drains. The retinaculi are sutured over the anterior tibial tendon unless the structures are extremely tight and the skin is good. After skin closure, a compression dressing is applied but no splint or cast is used unless an extremely unstable ankle is encountered.
17. Post-op care as previously described.

References

1. Cagoon, J.R., and Paxton, A.W.: A metallurgical survey of current orthopedic implants. *J. Biomed. Mater. Res.*, **4**:223–224, 1970.
2. Scholz, K.C.: Total Ankle Replacement Arthroplasty. In J.E. Bateman (Ed.): *Foot Science*, W.B. Saunders, Philadelphia, 1976.
3. Bateman, J.E. (Ed.): *Foot Science*, W.B. Saunders, Philadelphia, 1976, p. 109.
4. Thompson, P., Parkridge-Richards Laboratories: TPR Total Ankle. *Product Information Bulletin*, 1976.
5. Smith, R.C.: Smith Total Ankle Surgical Procedure. *Wright Laboratories Product Information Bulletin*, 1976.
6. Groth, H.: The Oregon Total Ankle. *Product Information Bulletin, Zimmer International*, Warsaw, In.

Selected Bibliography

Close, J.R.: Some application of the functional anatomy of the ankle joint. *J. Bone Jt. Surg.*, **38A**:761–781, 1956.

Isman, R.E., and Inman, V.T.: Anthropometric studies of the human foot and ankle. *Bull. Pros. Res.*, **10–11**:97–129, 1969.

Kempson, G.E., and Freeman, T.M.: Engineering consideration in the design of an ankle joint. *Biomech. Eng.*, 168, 1975.

Root, M.L., Orien, W.P., and Weed, J.H.: *Normal and Abnormal Function of the Foot*, Clinical Biomechanical Corporation, Los Angeles, 1978, pp. 181-290.

Sammorco, G.J., Burstein, A.H., and Frankel, V.H.: Biomechanics of the ankle: A kinematic study. *Orthoped. Clin. North Am.*, **4**:75–76, 1973.

Scales, J.T., and Lowe, S.A.: *Some Factors Influencing Bone and Joint Replacement*, J.B. Lippincott, Philadelphia, 1971.

Wright, D.G., DeSai, S.M., and Henderson, W.: Action of the subtalar and ankle complex during the stance phase of walking. *J. Bone Jt. Surg.*, **46A**:361–382, 1964.

CHAPTER 16

Reconstructive Procedures for Medial and Lateral Ankle Instability

To stabilize an ankle weakened by rupture of the lateral ligaments, or by acute injury to the talofibular or talocalcaneal ligaments, it is possible to restructure damage with the peroneus brevis tendon. Before any such operative approach is contemplated, however, conservative treatment should be attempted. In the case of severe, intractable instability, documented roentgenographically, corrective surgery is the treatment of choice.

In the case of lateral instability, both the Watson-Jones[1] and the Evans[2] techniques are commonly employed. The Watson-Jones technique restores function of the calcaneofibular and the talofibular ligaments by rerouting the peroneus brevis tendon. The chief drawback of this procedure is that it involves drilling a hole through the neck of the talus, a difficult task to accomplish with accuracy. A second major difficulty can arise with this technique if the peroneus brevis is too short to be threaded through the tunnels fashioned to receive it. The Evans technique, which was designed to obviate the potential difficulties of the Watson-Jones technique, has the disadvantage that it involves reconstruction of only the calcaneofibular ligament.

Other procedures commonly used for repair of lateral ankle instability include the Nilsonne, Lee, Elmslie, and the Chrisman and Snook technique. The procedure described by Dr. Harold Nilsonne[3] consisted of a tendonosis of the peroneal brevis tendon into the fibula along with repair of the inferior calcaneal fibular ligament. The Lee procedure[4] is also a tendonosis, threading a full portion of the peroneal brevis tendon through an osseous drill hole in the fibular malleolus.

The Elmslie procedure[5] and the Chrisman and Snook technique,[6] were designed to repair the anterior talofibular and inferior calcaneofibular ligaments; the latter technique a method for preservation of peroneus brevis function.

The Schoolfield[7] and DuVries[8] procedures were designed to repair injury to the deltoid ligament, usually created by forced eversion with associated fracture of the medial malleolus. In both procedures the surgical approach to the deltoid ligament is similar; however, the DuVries procedure depends upon scarring of the ligament to maintain correction.

Watson-Jones Technique[9]

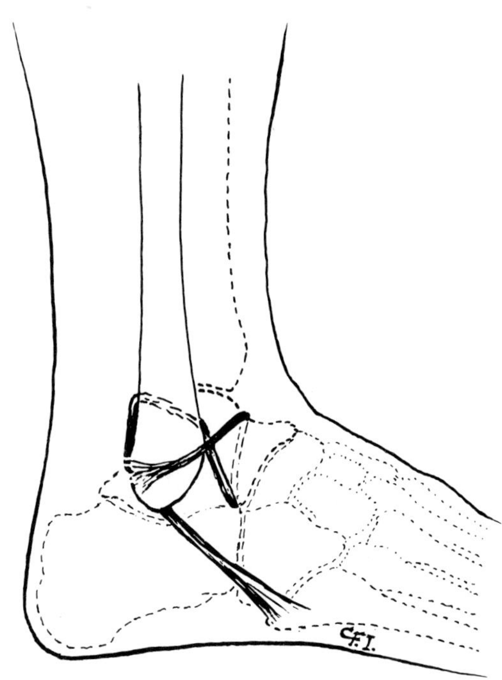

Figure 1. Modified Watson-Jones technique. (Reproduced with permission from Crenshaw, A.H. (Ed.): *Campbell's Operative Orthopaedics,* Vol. 1, C.V. Mosby, St. Louis, 1971, p. 945.)

1. Make a lateral incision over the ankle beginning proximally at the junction of the middle and distal thirds of the fibular shaft and continuing distally along the anterior border of the shaft. At this point, curve it anteriorly, and end 2 inches anterior to the tip of the lateral malleolus.
2. Divide the peroneus tendon as far proximally as possible from the muscle.
3. Suture the free end of the muscle to the peroneus longus tendon.
4. Free the peroneus brevis tendon as far distally as the lateral malleolus, leaving the peroneal retinacular intact.
5. Drill two tunnels through bone as follows.
   a. First drill a tunnel in an oblique anterior posterior direction through the lateral malleolus about 1 inch proximal to its tip.
   b. Drill a second tunnel in the longitudinal axis of the leg through the lateral part of the neck of talus, just anterior to the talofibular joint; it is easier to drill a hole in the superior lateral margin of the neck and another in the interolateral margin so that they join to form the tunnel.
6. Guide the peroneus brevis tendon through the first tunnel posteriorly to anteriorly, and through the second inferiorly to superiorly.
7. Unroll the remainder of the tendon to make it flat, and carry it posteriorly across the lateral surface of the malleolus after making an oblique incision through the periosteum at this level.

8. Suture the tendon to itself and to the periosteum on the posterior aspect of the malleolus. Then suture the periosteum to the tendon on the lateral side of the malleolus.
9. A short leg cast is applied for eight weeks. After the second or third week the cast is adjusted to permit walking.

Evans Procedure[9]

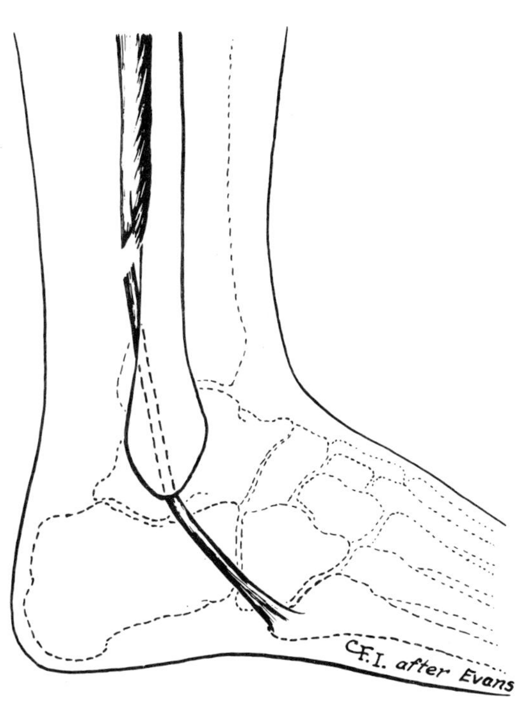

Figure 2. Evans technique. (Reproduced with permission from Crenshaw, A.H. (Ed.): *Campbell's Operative Orthopaedics*, Vol. 1, C.V. Mosby, St. Louis, 1971, p. 945.)

1. Approach, divide, and mobilize the peroneus brevis tendon as described above in the Watson-Jones technique.
2. Suture the free end of the peroneus brevis muscle to the peroneus longus tendon.
3. Drill a tunnel large enough to receive the tendon, beginning at the tip of the fibula and exiting posteriorly 1¼ inches proximal to the fibular tip.
4. Guide the tendon through the tunnel inferiorly to superiorly and suture it under tension to the adjacent soft tissue at both ends of the tunnel.
5. Apply a short leg cast for eight weeks; after three weeks, alter the cast for walking.

Lee's Modified Tenodesis[8]

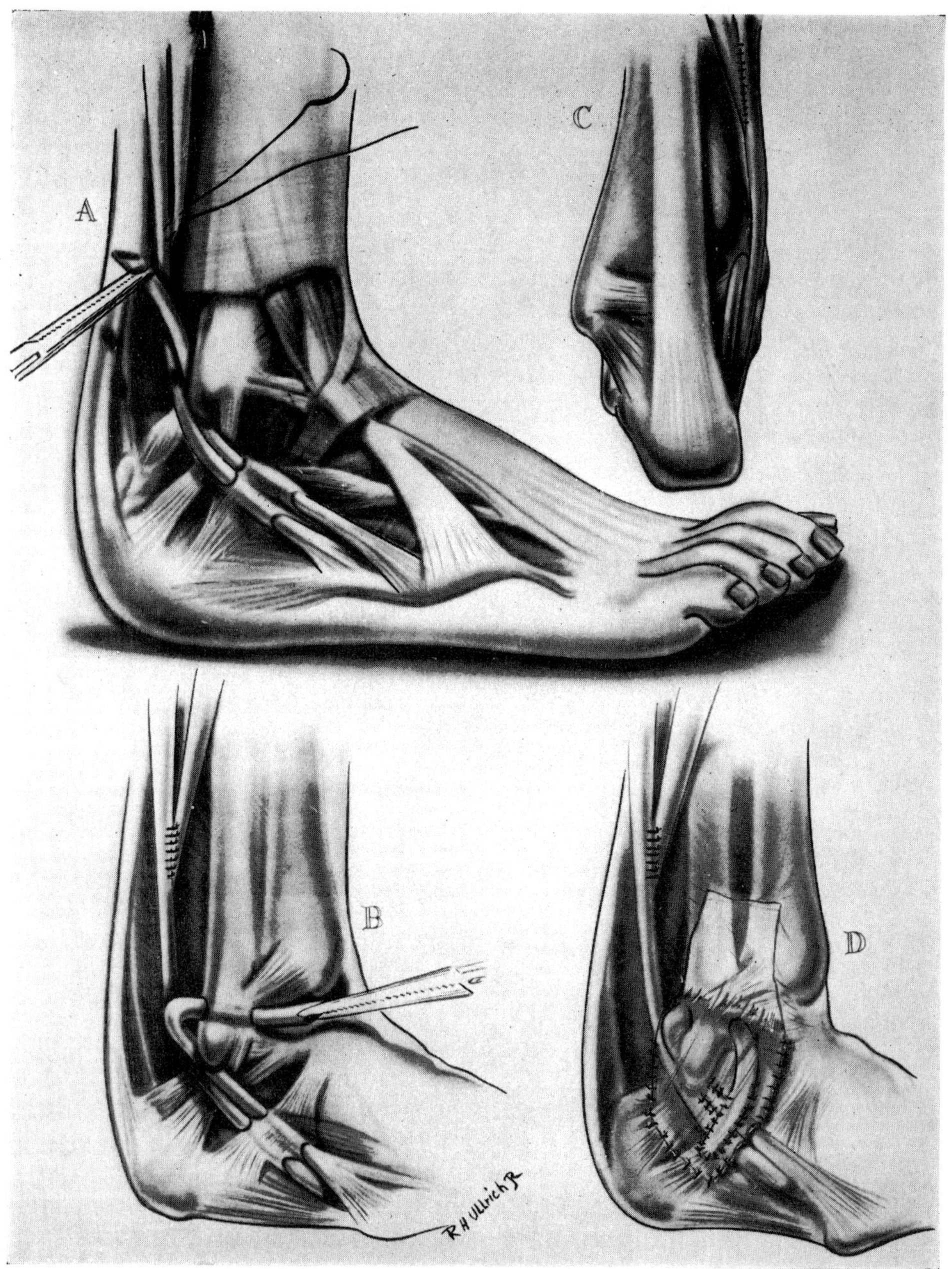

Figure 3. Lee's tenodesis for stabilization of the ankle. (A) Stripping of the peroneus brevis tendon. (B) Sutured proximal end of the peroneus brevis to the peroneus longus: Distal end of the peroneus brevis tendon guided through a drill hole in the lateral malleolus. (C) Posterior view. (D) Distal end of the peroneus brevis tendon sutured to itself and to the peroneus longus sheath, covered with a flap of fascia stripped from the malleolus. (Reproduced with permission from Lee, H.G.: *J. Bone & Joint Surg.* **39A**:828–833, 1957.)

1. Make a hockey-stick incision, beginning behind the lower third of the fibula, downward and around the lateral malleolus, and ending at the calcaneocuboid joint.
2. Incise the fascia, exposing the peroneal tendons.
3. Strip the peroneus brevis from its muscle belly as high as possible to obtain sufficient length to form a long loop through the malleolus.
4. Suture the loose muscle fibers of the peroneus brevis to the aponeurosis of the peroneus longus.
5. Free the peroneus brevis tendon down to the superior peroneal retinaculum, taking care not to disturb the ligamentous fibers.
6. Drill a horizontal hole ¼ inch in diameter, just below the broadest part of the lateral malleolus.
7. Thread the peroneus brevis tendon through the hole from back to front while the foot is held everted in correct valgus position, and draw the tendon downward, below the lateral malleolus. There, suture the tendon to itself and to the sheath of the peroneus longus.
8. Denude a flap of fascia from the lower portions of the fibula and tibia, fold the flap downward, and suture it to the surrounding tissues.
9. Apply a short leg cast for eight weeks; readjust after three weeks for walking.

Nilsonne Procedure[10]

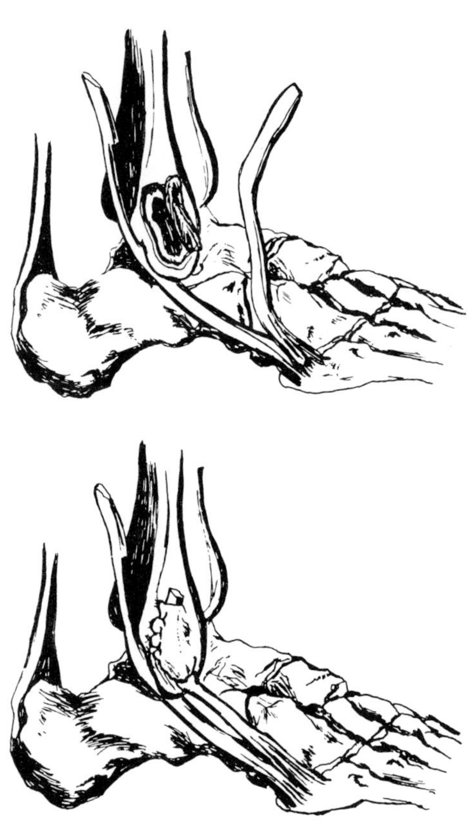

Figure 4. (Reproduced with permission from Zang, K.: *Traumatic Ankle Conditions,* Futura Publishing Company, Inc., Mt. Kisco, N.Y., 1976, p. 105.)

1. Make an incision parallel to the peroneal tendons that curve behind and below the fibular malleolus.
2. Expose and incise the superficial fascia down to the peroneus brevis tendon and separate it from its muscle fibers.
3. Divide the tendon transversely at the level of the superior retinaculum, and suture the proximal stump of the brevis to the longus.
4. Align the talocrural joint and create a groove subperiosteally in the lateral aspect of the fibular malleolus.
5. The ruptured inferior fibulocalcaneal ligament is then sutured together, and the distal portion of the peroneus brevis tendon is placed in the fibular groove and sutured.
6. The wound is closed in layers, and a short leg cast is applied.

Elmslie Procedure[10]

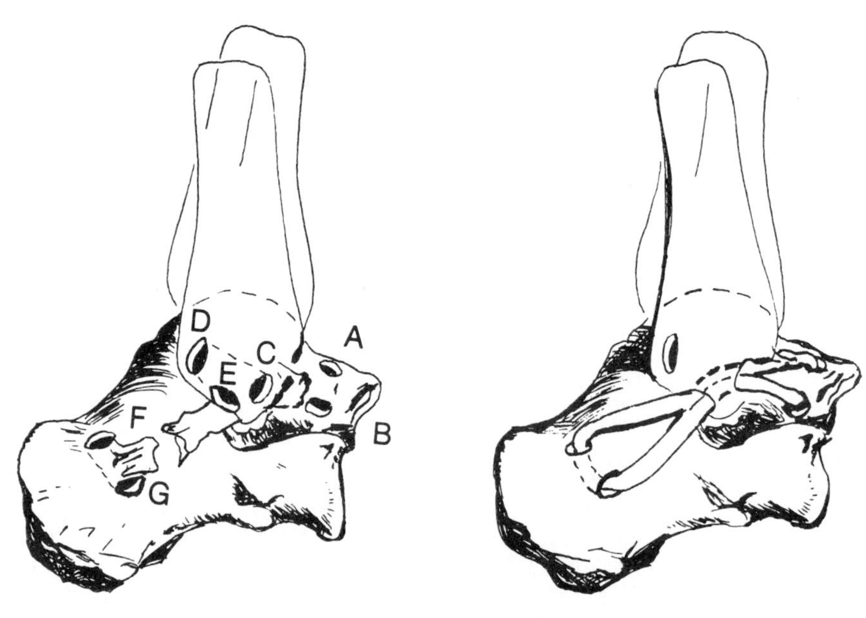

Figure 5. (Reproduced with permission from Zang, K.: *Traumatic Ankle Conditions*, Futura Publishing Company, Inc., Mt. Kisco, N.Y., 1976, p. 107.)

1. Make a curved incision approximately 5 inches long in a course parallel to the peroneal brevis tendon. Begin the incision 2 inches above the fibular malleolus and end midway between the malleolus and the base of the fifth metatarsal.
2. Reflect the skin, and deepen the incision anterior to the peroneal tendons down to bone. Retract the peroneal tendons inferiorly out of the wound.
3. The lateral surfaces of the talus, fibular malleolus, and calcaneus are exposed. Into the neck of talus, external malleolus and calcaneus, make a series of drill holes large enough to accept a cinch made of fascia lata.

4. A strip of fascia lata is then removed from the outer aspect of the thigh. The strip is approximately 8 inches long and ½ inch wide.
5. Thread the fascia through the various osseous tunnels to create a cinch.
6. The foot is then placed in a functional position at right angles and slight eversion, and the ends of the fascial strip are pulled tight and sutured with nonabsorbable material.
7. Wound closed in layers and short leg cast applied for eight weeks; after three weeks, adjust cast for walking.

Chrisman and Snook Procedure[10]

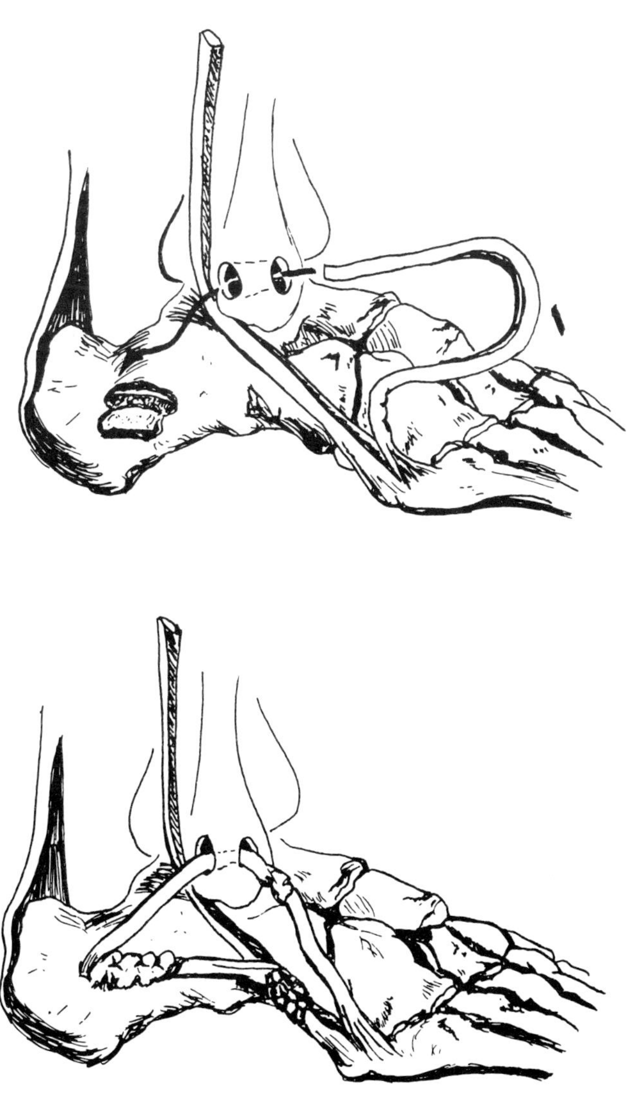

Figure 6. (Reproduced with permission from Zang, K.: *Traumatic Ankle Conditions*, Futura Publishing Company, Inc., Mt. Kisco, N.Y., 1976, p. 110.)

1. Incision proceeds distally to the posterior and inferior portion of the fibular malleolus. At this junction it continues to the base of the fifth metatarsal.
2. Deepen and expose the peroneus brevis tendon, which is split into an anterior and posterior portion from its insertion into the base of the fifth metatarsal up to its muscle belly.
3. The anterior portion of the the tendon is then freed from its muscle belly and is pulled distally from under the retinaculum. The split tendon is sectioned at its most proximal portion.
4. Concentrating on the talus, fibular malleolus and calcaneus, make a periosteal groove on the neck of the talus and lateral aspect of the calcaneus. At this point make an osseous tunnel through the fibula in the horizontal plane, approximately 1 inch proximal to its tip.
5. The split portion of the tendon is then passed through the tunnel anteriorly to posteriorly and is then directed plantarly to the groove in the calcaneus.
6. The tendon is passed through the groove and directed distally to the fifth metatarsal, with the foot maintained in a neutral position and slight eversion.
7. Under tension, the tendon is then sutured in the talar groove, then at its points of entry and exit in the fibular tunnel and calcaneal groove. Finally, it is sutured to the peroneal tendon at the base of the fifth metatarsal.
8. The wound is closed in layers, and a short leg cast is applied for eight weeks; after three weeks, adjust the cast for walking.

DuVries Procedure[9]

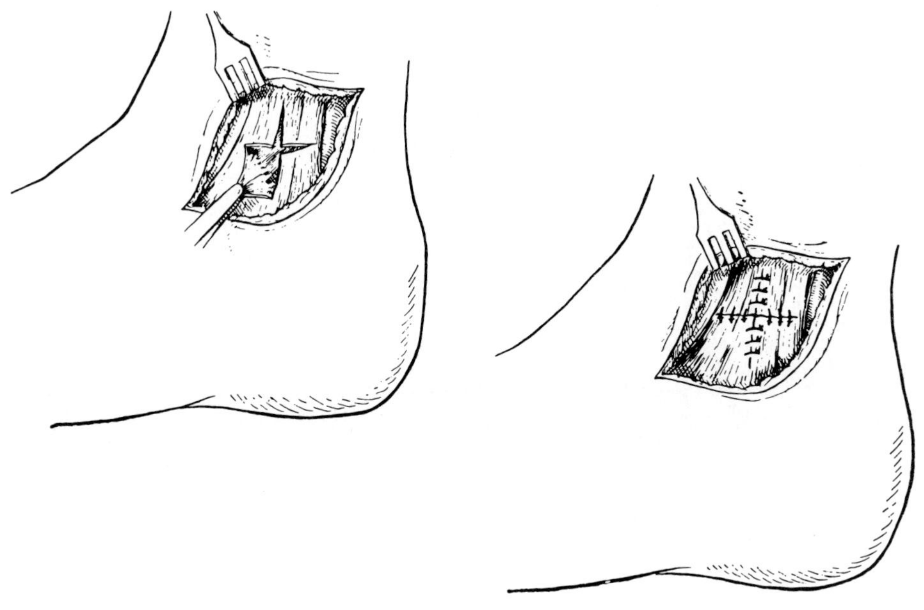

Figure 7. (Reproduced with permission from DuVries, H.L.: *Surgery of the Foot*, C.V. Mosby, St. Louis, 1959, p. 106.)

1. Make a curved incision over the medial aspect of the ankle beginning posterior to the medial malleolus, coursing distally and anteriorly about 2 cm distal to the malleolus, and ending over the tuberosity of the navicular.
2. Elevate the anterior skin flap and expose the deltoid ligament.
3. Make two incisions, one transverse and the other longitudinal, through the full thickness of the ligament to form a cross with equal arms.
4. Free the resulting four flaps of ligament from the underlying bone. Then suture the margins of the flaps together.
5. Apply a short leg cast for eight weeks; readjust the cast in three weeks for walking.

Schoolfield Technique[7]

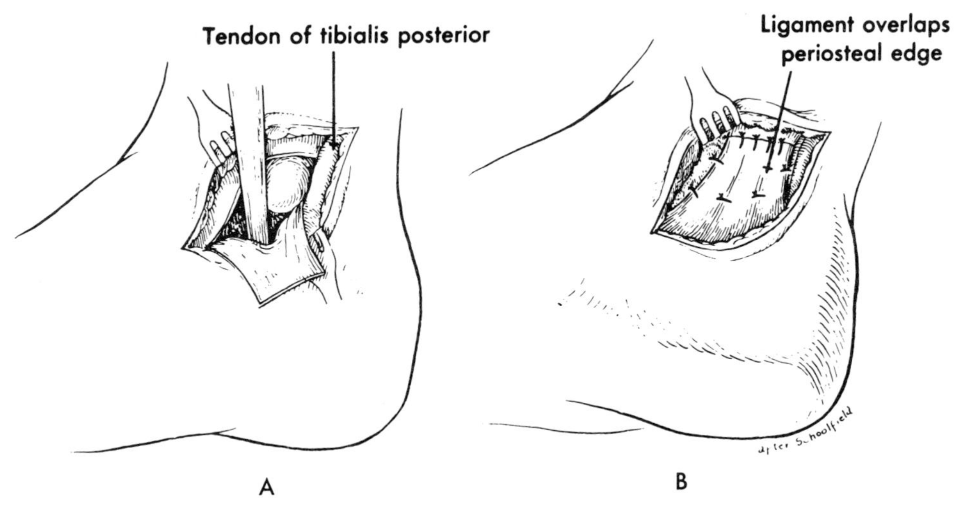

Figure 8. Schoolfield's technique. (A) Deltoid ligament stripped from above downward over the medical malleolus. (B) Foot held in inversion: Upper margin of the deltoid ligament is sutured to the periosteal edge, which it overlaps. (Reproduced with permission from Inman, V.T. (Ed.): *DuVries' Surgery of the Foot,* C.V. Mosby, St. Louis, 1973, p. 105.)

1. Make a semilunar incision, beginning behind the medial malleolus, coursing downward and curving anteriorly about 2 cm below the malleolus, and ending over the tuberosity of the navicular.
2. Deflect the anterior skin flap to expose the deltoid ligament, which is then detached from the medial malleolus and freed to its insertions.
3. Invert the foot to permit suturing of the deltoid ligament to the periosteal and ligamentous tissues over the medial malleolus, just above the natural origin of the deltoid ligament.
4. Apply a short leg cast with the foot held in inversion for eight weeks; readjust the cast in three weeks for walking.

References

1. Watson-Jones, R.: *Fractures and Joint Injuries*, 4 ed., Williams & Wilkins, Baltimore, 1952–1955.
2. Evans, D.L.: Recurrent instability of the ankle—A method of surgical treatment. *Proc. R. Soc. Med.*, **46**:343, 1953.
3. Nilsonne, A.: Making a new ligament in ankle sprain. *J. Bone Jt. Surg.*, **14**:380–381, 1932.
4. Lee, H.G.: Surgical repair in recurrent dislocation of the ankle joint. *J. Bone Jt. Surg.*, **35A**:828–833, 1957.
5. Elmslie, R.C.: Recurrent subluxations of the ankle joint. *Ann. Surg.*, **100**:364, 1934.
6. Chrisman and Snook: Reconstruction of the lateral ligaments of the ankle. *J. Bone Jt. Surg.*, **51-A**:904–1912, 1969.
7. Schoolfield, B.L.: Operative treatment of flatfoot. *Surg. Gynecol. & Obstet.* **94**:136–140, 1955.
8. DuVries, H: *Surgery of the Foot*, 2 ed., C.V. Mosby, St. Louis, 1959.
9. Crenshaw, A.H. (Ed.): *Campbell's Operative Orthopaedics*, Vols. 1 and 2, C.V. Mosby, St. Louis, 1971.
10. Zang, K.: *Traumatic Ankle Conditions*, Futura Publishing Company, Inc., Mt. Kisco, N.Y., 1976.

Selected Bibliography

Dziob, J.: Ligamentous injuries about the ankle joint. *Am. J. Surg.*, **91**:692, 1956.

Hambly, E.: Recurrent dislocation of the ankle due to rupture of external lateral ligament. *Br. Med. J.*, **1**:413, 1945.

Leonard, M.H.: Injuries of the lateral ligaments of the ankle. *J. Bone Jt. Surg.*, **31-A**:373, 1949.

Ruth, C.: The surgical treatment of injuries of the fibular collateral ligaments of the ankle. *J. Bone Jt. Surg.*, **43-A**:229, 1961.

Wilson, J.D.: Sprains and ruptures of ligaments of the ankle joint. In A.F. DePalma (Ed.): *Clinical Orthopaedics*, Vol. 3, J. B. Lippincott, Philadelphia, 1954.

CHAPTER 17

Tendon Transfers and the Paralytic Foot

Paralysis of the muscles of the lower leg and foot generally leads to lateral instability and a limited degree of dorsiflexion of the foot. In such cases operative correction is best if it is carried out early in childhood, before ossification occurs. The surgical approach generally involves tendon transfer to preserve contracture function and to prevent further atrophy of the muscles of the lower limb. Tendon transfer improves motor power and brings about greater joint stability. Before tendon transfer can be considered, however, the muscle or muscles involved in the paralysis must be evaluated for strength and for the feasibility of maintaining a straight line in the course of transfer. Furthermore, the transferred tendon must pass through smooth tissue so that it may move without restriction. Unless these three preoperative criteria can be met, operation for tendon transfer is contraindicated.

When the foot surgeon is faced with the possibility of tendon transfer, a complete muscle examination must be performed so that one can predict whether the transferred muscle will be capable of performing its new function. As some degree of strength is lost in muscle transfer, a rule of thumb to follow is not to utilize a muscle with a tested strength beneath a good to normal rating. As will be the case in any surgical procedure, exceptions will be encountered, as in the utilization of both the peroneus longus and brevis muscles, whose strength is considered fair on an individual basis, but whose combined transference may produce adequate dorsiflexor power in the absence of posterior calf muscle contracture. The surgeon is usually also put upon to decide as to the use of transference prior to, or after, the correction of existing deformity. Various authors expound the philosophy that deformity must be corrected first. It has been our experience, however, that individuals in whom the growth period has not been exceeded will fare well if transference is performed with the purpose of diminishing the deforming forces and allowing the patient the chance of having optimal bony growth in an atmosphere of tendonous stability. If the deformity persists beyond the growth years, the surgeon may then perform the more radical arthrodesis procedure. It is also the responsibility of the surgeon to be aware of the many pitfalls of tendon transfer and the possibilities of abnormal foot function and new deformities which can be created. Of major concern to the operating surgeon, and probably the most neglected aspect of the surgery, is the re-education of the muscle. It is this postoperative training, which must be actively pursued, which can predispose the transference to success or failure.

I. Paralysis of the Evertor Muscles—Equinovarus

When the peroneus (evertor) muscles are paralyzed, calcaneal inversion results, because the action of the posterior tibial muscle goes unopposed. Forefoot varus then develops because the action of the anterior tibial muscle also is unopposed. Over time, the varus deformity can lead to formation of dorsal bunion.

Technique for Correction[1]

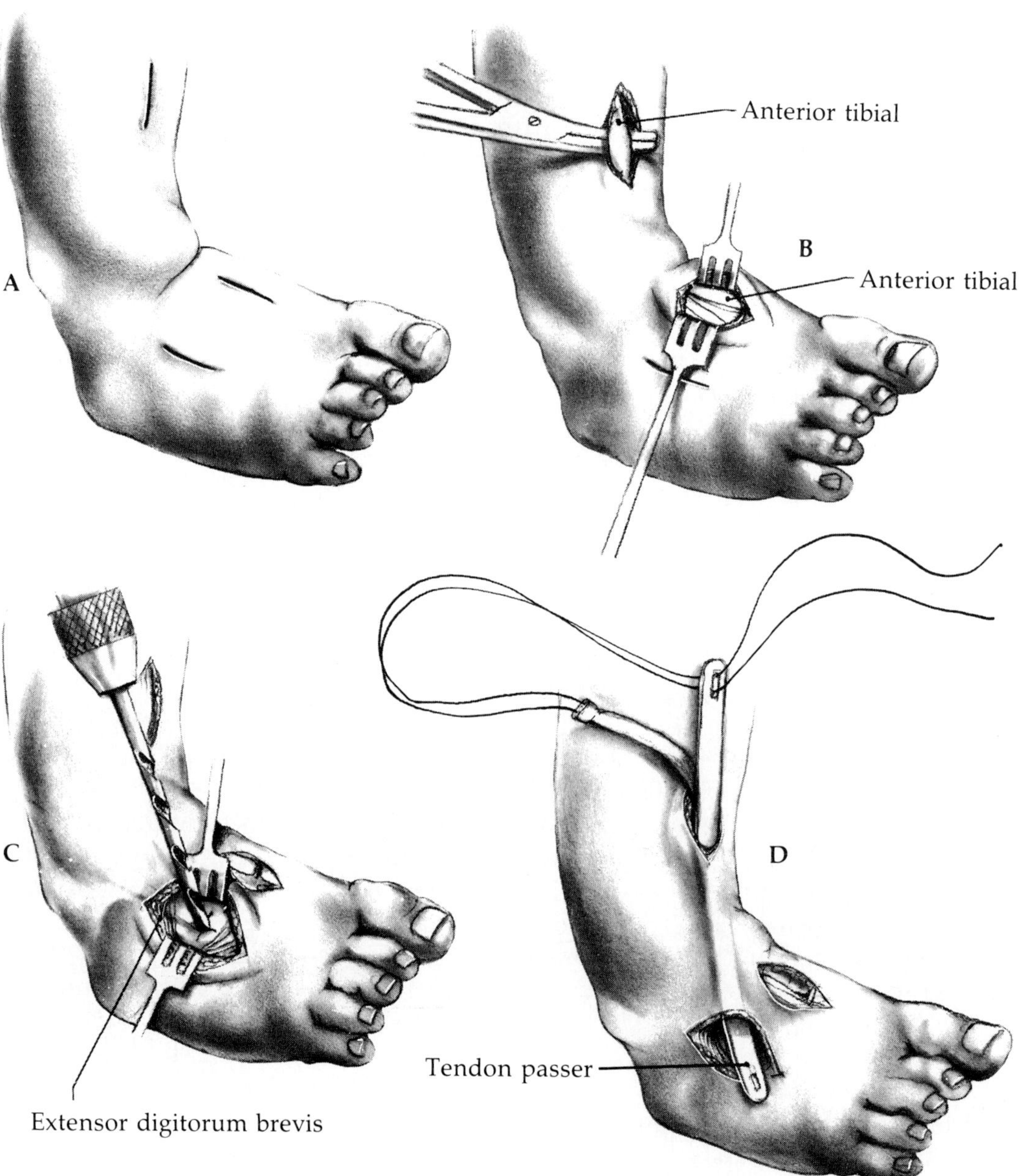

Figure 1. (Reproduced with permission from Goldstein, L.A., and Dickerson, R.C.: *Atlas of Orthopaedic Surgery*, Vol. 2, C.V. Mosby, St. Louis, 1974, pp. 923, 925, 927.) *Continued on facing page.*

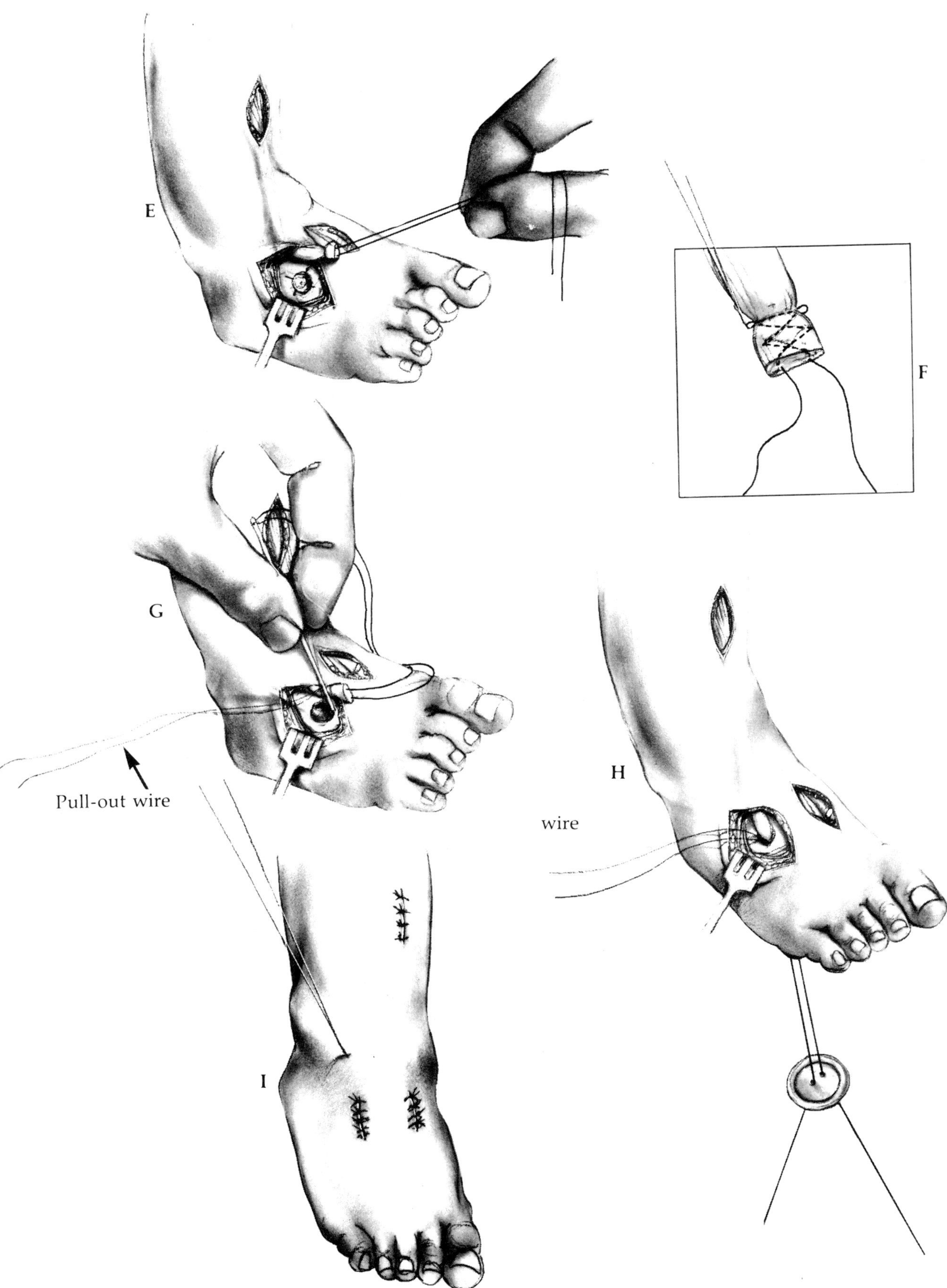
E
F
G
Pull-out wire
H
wire
I

1. Make three skin incisions, one over the dorsomedial aspect of the base of the first metatarsal, another 5 cm above the ankle, and a third over the internal cuneiform.
2. A subcutaneous tunnel is made with a clamp between the second and third incisions to prepare the tendon's new course. The insertion of the anterior tibial tendon is then detached as far distally as possible, together with a fascial tongue. The muscle–tendon structure is identified in the proximal incision. The tendon is then pulled through the leg incision and subsequently passed through the prepared tunnel to its new insertion point.
3. A drill hole is then made through the plantar aspect of the third cuneiform.
4. A pull-out, Bunnell, stainless steel suture is placed in the transferred tendon. The two ends of the Bunnell suture are then passed through the drill hole in the plantar aspect of the foot.
5. The tendon is pulled securely into the bony bed, and the wire suture is tied over a small gauze pad and button on the plantar aspect of the foot, with the foot held in mild valgus and the ankle in neutral.
6. The pull-out suture is then passed through the skin and the wounds are closed.
7. The foot is held in mild valgus, and immobilization in a plaster cast is continued for six weeks.

II. Paralysis of Peroneal, Extensor Digitorum Longus, and Extensor Hallucis Longus—Equinovarus

When the peroneals, the extensor digitorum longus, and the hallucis longus muscles are weak, a mild equinovarus will result. In order to restore proper balance, the tibialis anticus must be transferred laterally to the base of the third metatarsal.

Technique for Correction

Lateral transfer of the tibialis anticus, as described above.

III. Paralysis of the Invertor Muscles—Planovalgus

Weakness of the anterior tibial muscle will cause a loss of dorsiflexion-inversion power in the absence of an equinus; however, in the presence of an equinus they will be unable to take over the action of the tibialis anticus. The proximal phalanges of the toes become hyperextended and depress the metatarsal heads, causing cock-up toe deformities. Occasionally, cavovarus deformity of the foot may result because of the action of the peroneus longus muscle which acts as a depressor of the first metatarsal.

Technique for Correction[1]

Transfer of the peroneus longus muscle.

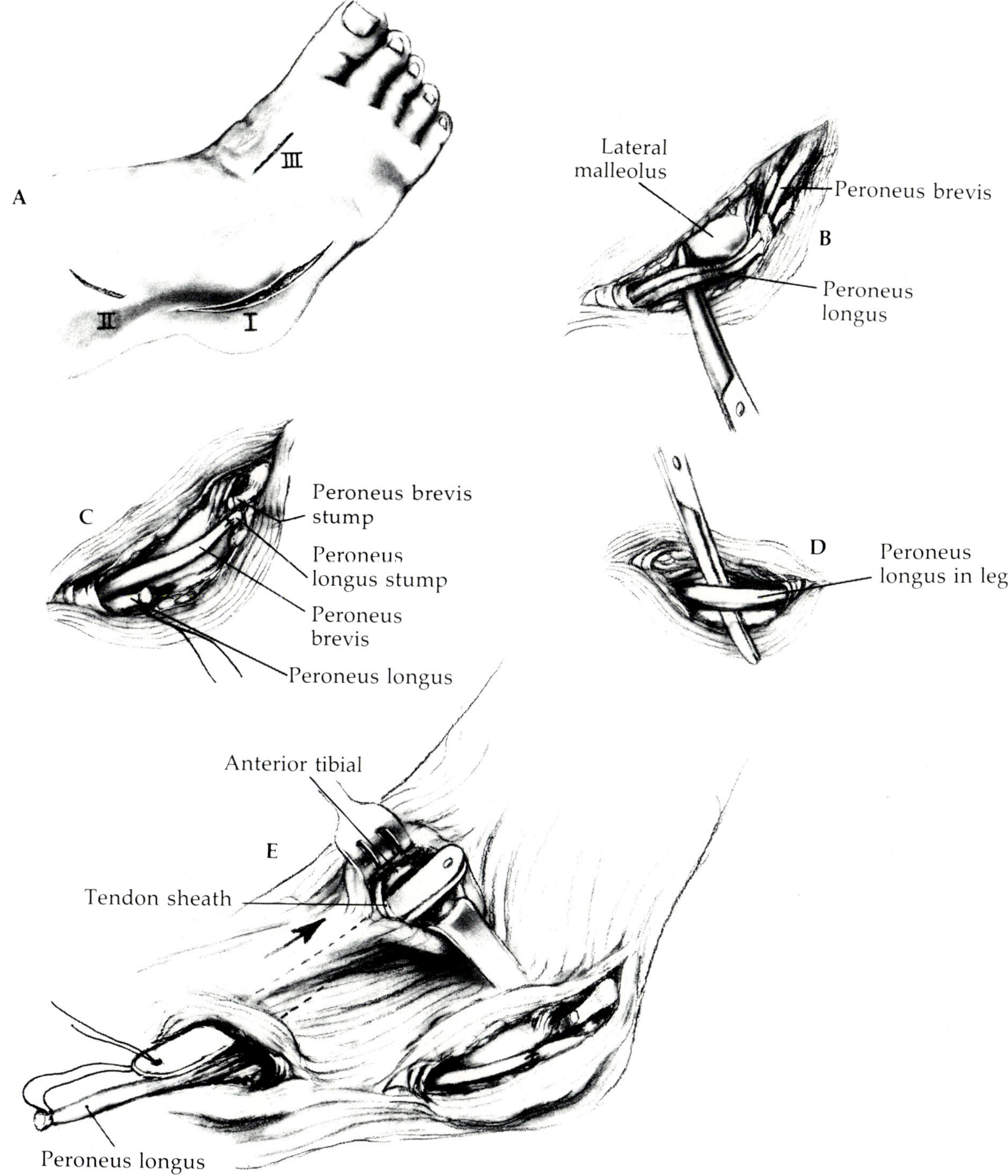

Figure 2. (Reproduced with permission from Goldstein, L.A., and Dickerson, R.C.: *Atlas of Orthopaedic Surgery,* Vol. 2, C.V. Mosby, St. Louis, 1974, pp. 919, 921.) *Continued on next page.*

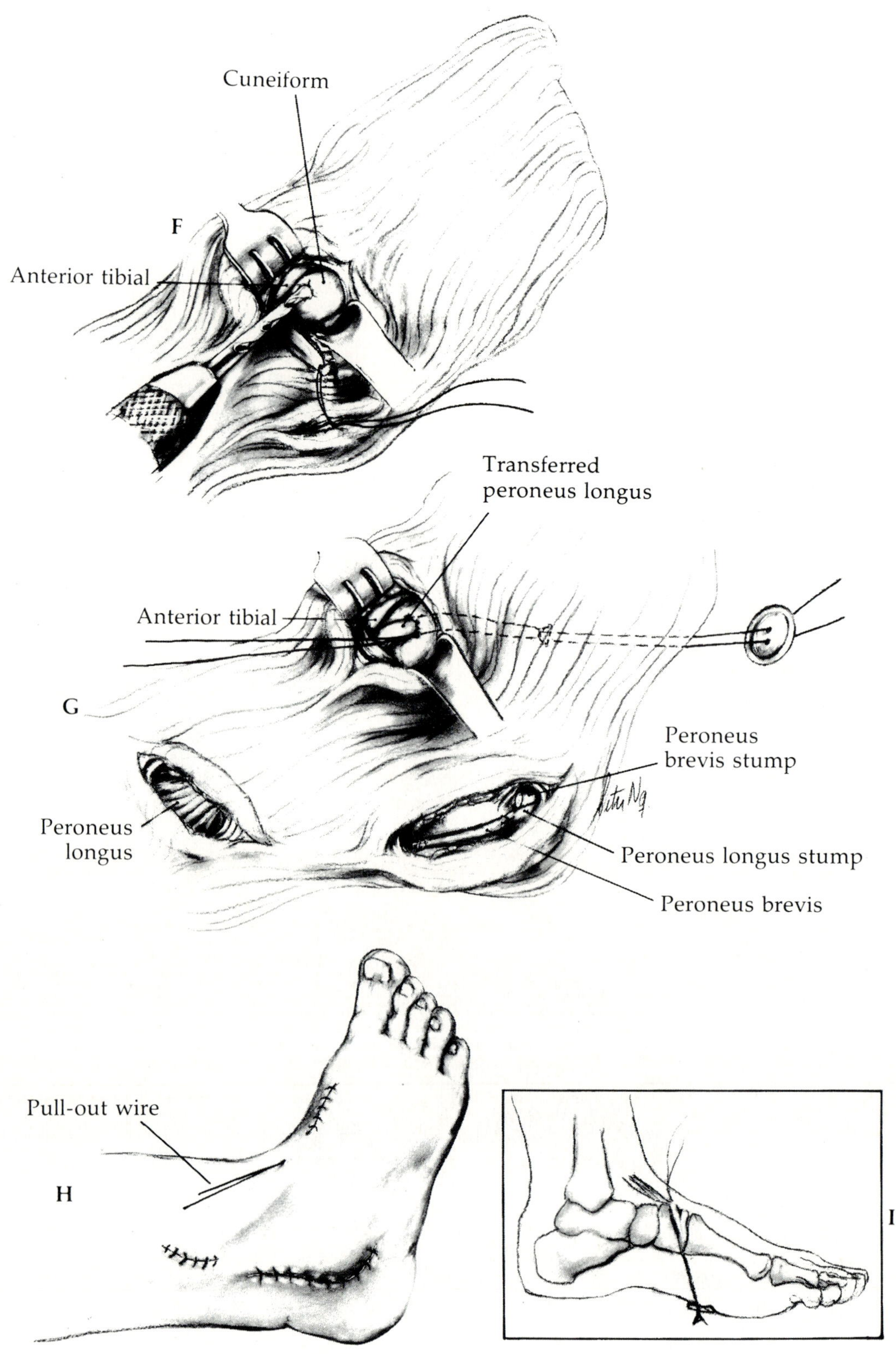

Figure 2 (continued). (Reproduced with permission from Goldstein, L.A., and Dickerson, R.C.: *Atlas of Orthopaedic Surgery*, Vol. 2, C.V. Mosby, St. Louis, 1974, pp. 919, 921.)

1. Three skin incisions are made.
   a. The first is made over the lateral aspect of the leg at the musculotendinous junction of the peroneus longus muscle. The lateral sural compartment is opened and the tendon of the peroneus longus identified and separated from the brevis.
   b. The second is made on the lateral plantar aspect of the cuboid. The longus tendon is identified and followed well underneath the cuboid. Then the peroneus longus tendon is severed as far underneath the foot as possible.
   c. The third is made on the dorsum of the foot. Usually placement is over the base of the second metatarsal; however, if the tibialis anticus is completely paralyzed, the incision is made over the base of the first metatarsal. The incision is then deepened to bone, and a drill hole is made from dorsal to plantar to receive the tendon.
2. The peroneus longus tendon is then drawn proximally out of the wound through the lateral leg incision.
3. A uterine packing forcep is then passed retrograde from the dorsum of the foot through the superficial plane beneath the cruciate ligaments to the lateral aspect of the anterior muscle compartment. The intermuscular septum dividing the anterior and lateral compartments is perforated, and the tip of the forceps is passed into the lateral compartment. A Dexon® suture is placed into the tip of the tendon, and the two ends of the suture are grasped by the tip of the forceps. The forceps is withdrawn, and the suture is used to draw the peroneus longus distally to the dorsum of the foot. The tendon should be transferred without excessive tension.
4. Two Keith needles are then attached to the tips of the Dexon® suture, and the suture is pulled through the drill hole to the plantar aspect of the foot and tied over a well-padded button.
5. Closure of the wounds should be meticulous, especially the deep fascia over the peroneal muscles, to prevent herniation.
6. The foot is then placed in a short leg walking cast for six weeks.
7. A night splint may be beneficial following cast removal to maintain a stretching of the posterior muscles, as well as to allow the peroneus longus to contract and adjust to its ideal functional length.

IV. Paralysis of the Anterior Tibial, Toe Extensors, and Peroneals—Equinovarus

Although preservation of the dorsiflexion function of the foot is not a primary objective of rehabilitation (it can be controlled by bracing), its restoration is generally helpful and should be accomplished whenever possible. When the action of the soleus, the gastrocnemius, and the posterior tibial muscles goes unopposed, as in cerebral palsy, an equinovarus deformity results. Correction can be accomplished by the Ober procedure for anterior transfer of the posterior tibial tendon.

Technique for Correction[2]

Anterior transfer of posterior tibial tendon. Ober technique.

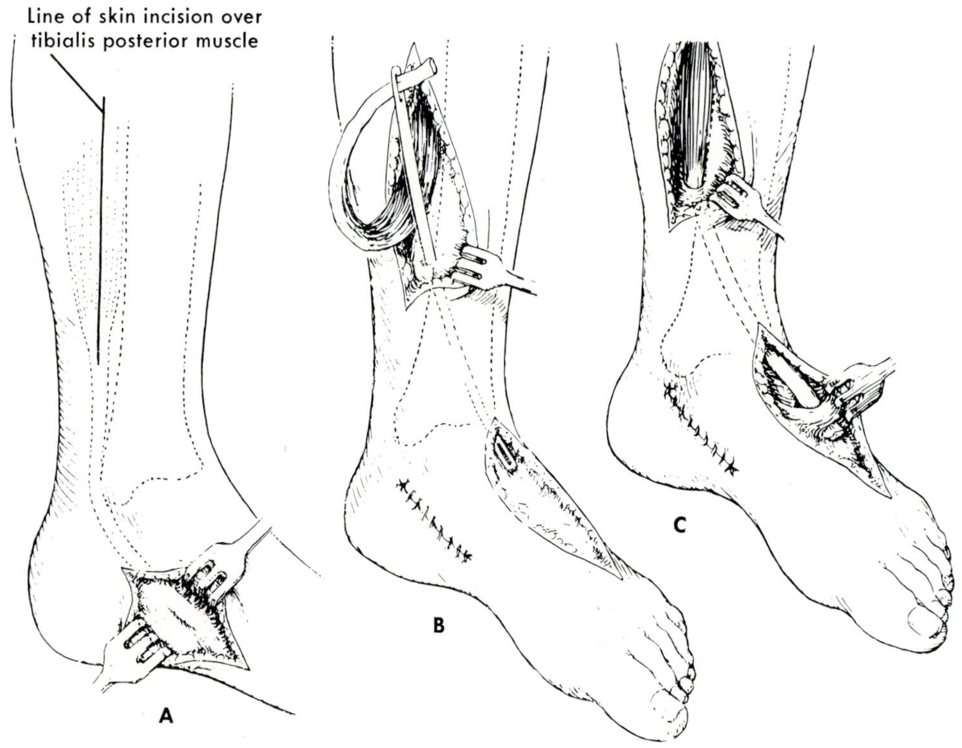

Figure 3. Ober anterior transfer of tibialis posterior tendon. (A) Insertion of tibialis posterior tendon has been exposed. Note line of skin incision over muscle. (B) Tendon has been freed from its insertion and muscle has been dissected from tibia. (C) Tendon and muscle have been passed through anterior tibial compartment to dorsum of foot, and tendon has been anchored in third metatarsal. (Redrawn from Ober, F.R.: *New Eng. J. Med.* **209**:52, 1933. Reproduced with permission from Crenshaw, A.H. (Ed.): *Campbell's Operative Orthopaedics*, Vol. 2, C.V. Mosby, St. Louis, 1971, p. 1557.)

1. Make an incision approximately 3 inches in length, in a medial longitudinal fashion, and free the attachment of the tibialis posterior tendon to the navicular.
2. Make a second incision over the musculotendinous junction of the tibialis posterior, also in a medial longitudinal fashion.
3. Through the proximal incision, withdraw the tendon and free the muscle up along the tibia.
4. Remove the periosteum in an oblique direction across the medial aspect of the tibia, such that when the tendon is transposed to the anterior compartment, only muscle belly will contact denuded bone. The tendon must never contact the tibia.
5. Now make a third incision into the base of the third metatarsal, and pull the

tibialis posterior tendon from the proximal leg incision into the third incision; at this point anchor the tendon into the base of the third metatarsal.

6. Long leg cast is applied for six weeks, bivalving at three weeks with rehabilitative exercises begun.
7. The transfer is then protected for six months by a double bar drop foot brace with an outside T-strap.

V. Paralysis of the Plantar Flexors—Calcaneus Deformity

Paralysis of the plantar flexors is most often associated with poliomyelitis and myelomeningococel. This disability causes weakness of the triceps surae, which leads to upward displacement of the talar head and the body weight to the tibia and resultant dorsiflexion of the ankle joint. A calcaneal limp is usually evident.

Technique for Correction

Posterior transfers. Since the triceps surae are the strongest muscles of the foot, it is advisable to transfer three or four muscles posteriorly to the calcaneus. The best results of tendon transfer are found when there is only partial loss of the gastrocnemius–soleus function. When there is complete loss of the triceps surae, a fairly good gait can be obtained by transferring the posterior tibial, the flexor hallucis longus, and both peroneal tendons. In such a case arthrodesis is necessary to prevent instability.

References

1. Goldstein, L.A., and Dickerson, R.C.: *Atlas of Orthopaedic Surgery*, Vol. 2, C.V. Mosby, St. Louis, 1974.
2. Crawford, A.H.: A Discussion of Tendon Transfers. *Arch. Pod. Med. Foot Surg.*, **II**:47–60, 1974.

Selected Bibliography

Crenshaw, A.H. (Ed.): *Campbell's Operative Orthopaedics*, Vol. 2, C.V. Mosby, St. Louis, 1963.

Hoffer, M.M.: The split anterior tibial tendon transfer of spastic varus hindfoot. *Orthoped. Clin. North Am.*, 5**(1)**, 1974.

Mayer, I.: The physiological method of tendon transplantation. *Surg. Gynecol. Obstet.*, **22**:182, 1916.

McGlamry, E.D.: *Reconstructive Surgery of the Foot and Leg*, Intercontinental Medical Book Corp., New York, 1974.

Ober, F.R.: Tendon transplantation in the lower extremity. *N. Eng. J. Med.*, **209**:52, 1933.

Turner, J.W., and Cooper, R.R.: Posterior transposition of the tibialis anterior through the interosseous membrane. *Clin. Orthoped. Relat. Res.* **79**:71–74, 1971.

Westin, G.W.: Tendon transfers about the foot, ankle, and hip in the paralyzed lower extremity. *J. Bone Jt. Surg.*, **47-A**:1430–1443, 1965.

CHAPTER 18

Soft Tissue Procedures in the Correction of Clubfoot

The residual varus deformity of clubfoot has long been corrected by medial release of excessive soft tissue contracture. The objective of the many procedures developed for this purpose is to release posterior, medial, or subtalar muscle and ligament contractures. Posterior tightening may relate to the posterior capsule of the ankle and subtalar joints, the tendo Achillis, and the posterior talofibular and calcaneofibular ligaments. Medial contractures involve the deltoid and spring ligaments, the talonavicular capsule, and several tendons, including the posterior tibial, the flexor digitorum longus, and the flexor hallucis longus. Subtalar contracture involves the anterior interosseous ligament on the bifurcate ligament.

The Dickerson and Goldstein[1] and the Gelman[2] techniques were developed to deal with posterior contractures. The Bost[3] technique is used to correct medial contractures, and Turco[4] developed a procedure by which all soft tissue contractures can be corrected at once. Garceau's technique[5] is appropriate when several elements of contracture deformity have recurred and when the peroneus longus and brevis muscles are weakened or absent. It is also employed in correction of supination of the forefoot during the swing phase of gait.

The correction of all of the elements of clubfoot is also advocated by Tachdjian, who for the most part concurs with Turco that a posterior release is not sufficient to correct the entire deformity of a talipis equino varus. Both authors are of the opinion that the varus component of the calcaneus must be considered, and, as such, the calcaneus and navicular must be released in combination with a posterior release. Turco, in an effort to sustain correction achieved through surgery and commonly lost by use of plaster of Paris immobilization alone, was initially responsible for advocating a procedure of transfixing the talonavicular joint with a thin Kirschner wire. Tachdjian, although agreeing in theory with Turco, has modified his procedure by making a longitudinal incision on the medial aspect of the tendo calcaneus, thus increasing surgical exposure. Tachdjian, secondly, alters his medial incision by making it perpendicular to the fixed inverted position of the everted heel, thereby approximating the wound edges more correctly. A final modification incorporated by Tachdjian is the placement of a Steinmann pin through the lateral side to maintain the equinus correction.

Techniques involving posterior tibial tendon transfer after correction of clubfoot are becoming more and more popular. This approach can be helpful only when the contracture deformities have been repaired. The tendon transfer procedures are detailed in Chapter 17.

Dickerson and Goldstein Technique[1]

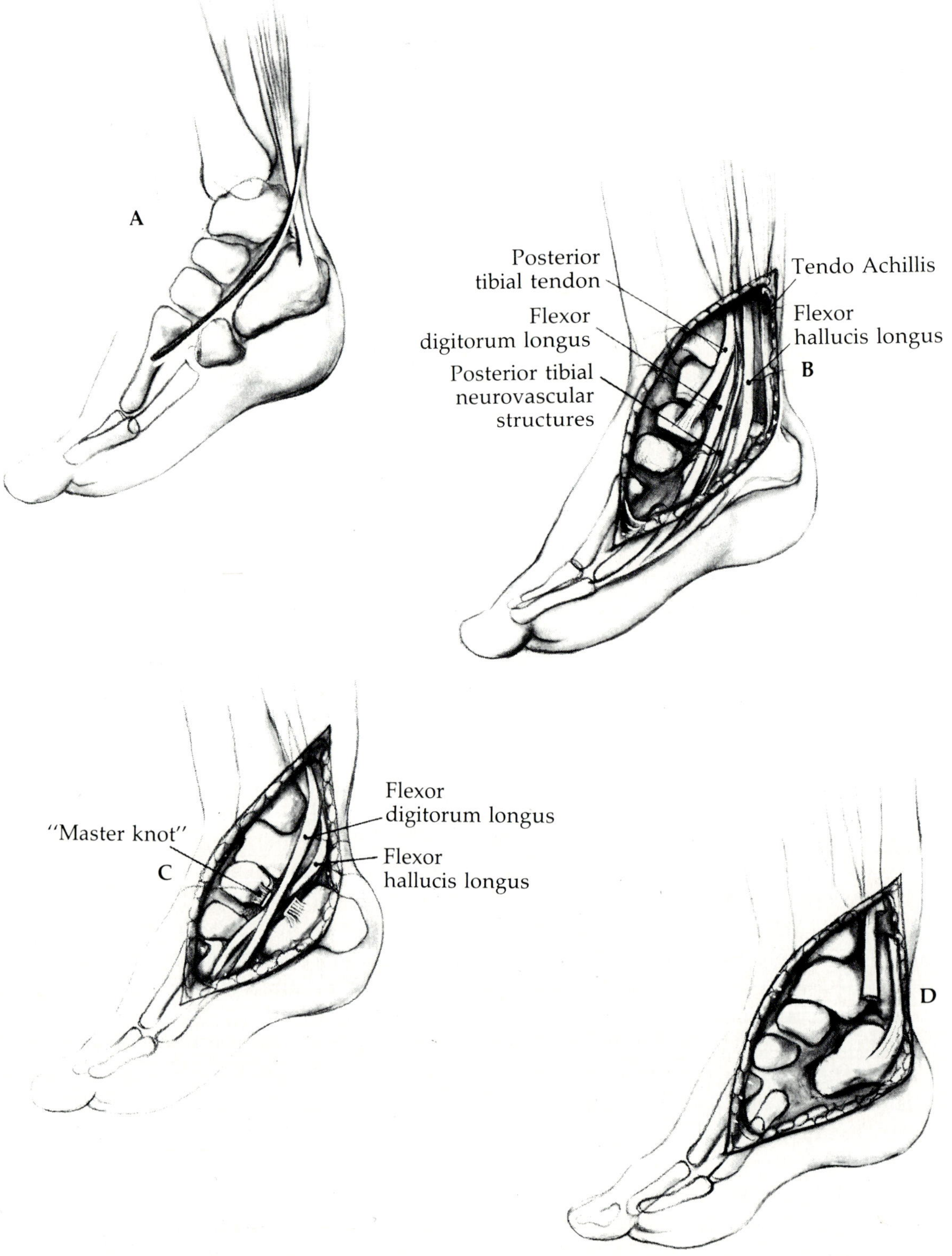

Figure 1. (Reproduced with permission from Goldstein, L.A., and Dickerson, R.C.: *Atlas of Orthopaedic Surgery*, Vol. 2, C.V. Mosby, St. Louis, 1974, pp. 913, 915.) *Continued on facing page.*

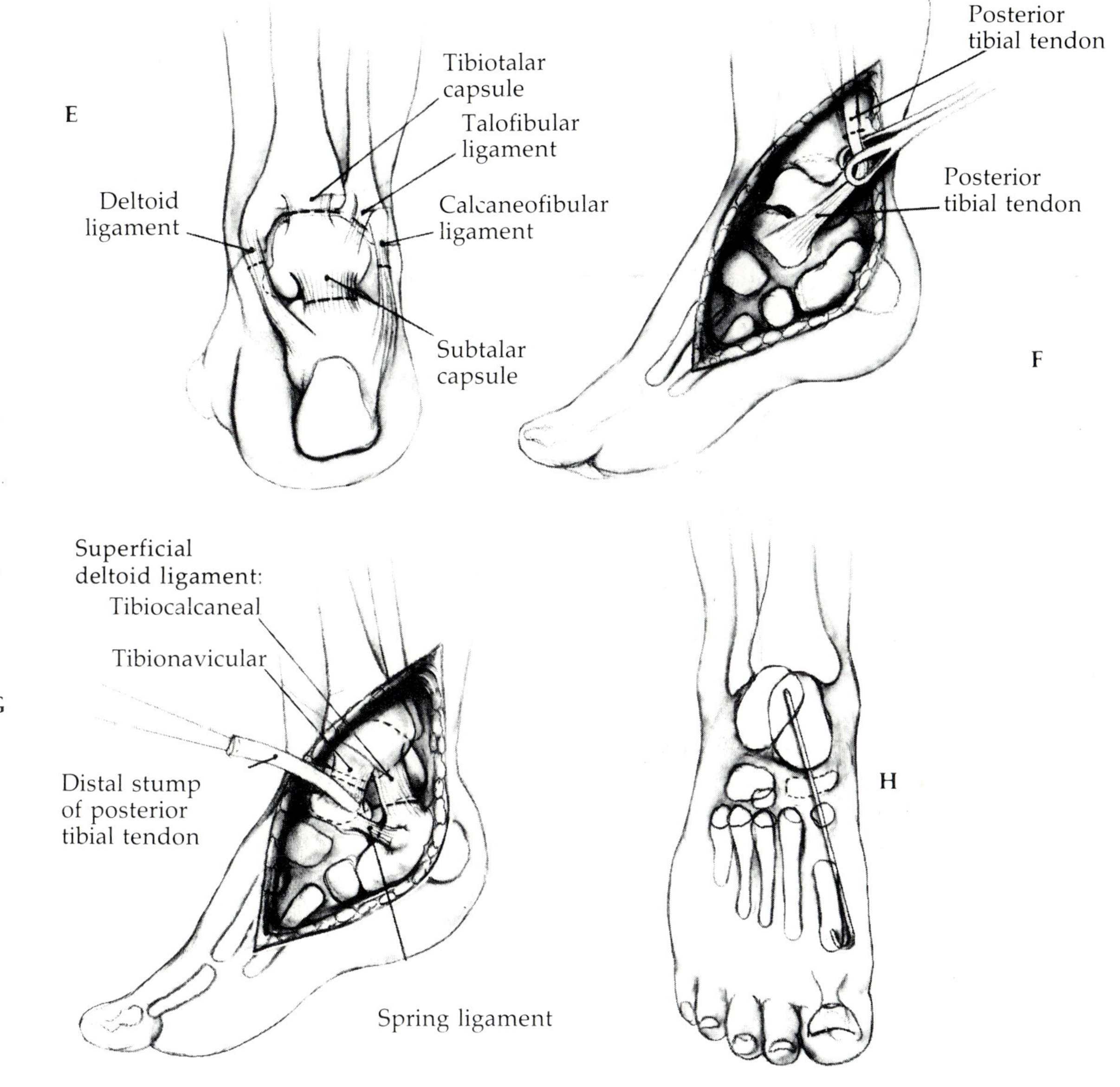

Figure 1 (continued). (Reproduced with permission from Goldstein, L.A., and Dickerson, R.C.: *Atlas of Orthopaedic Surgery*, Vol. 2, C.V. Mosby, St. Louis, 1974, pp. 913, 915.)

1. A 9 cm incision beginning at the first metatarsal and continuing posteriorly to the Achilles tendon, curving slightly under the medial malleolus.
2. Expose and open the sheaths at the posterior tibial tendon, flexor digitorum longus, flexor hallucis longus and the tendo Achillis.
3. Once the sheaths are open the next step is to mobilize the navicular. The flexor hallucis longus tendon's sheaths must be freed by dividing the "Master Knot" of Henry. (This is a fibrocartilagenous structure that at-

taches under the navicular and encompasses the flexor digitorum longus and flexor hallucis longus tendons as they cross.)

4. Now excise the soft tissue contracture. The posterior release must be done first to facilitate the incision at the medial and subtalar contractures.
5. Lengthen the Achilles tendon by Z-plasty, detaching the medial half from the calcaneus.
6. Identify the posterior margin of the tibia and perform a posterior capsulotomy.
7. Next transect the posterior talofibular ligament, the posterior capsule of the subtalar joint, the calcaneofibular ligament, and finally, retracting the neurovascular bundle posteriorly, divide the posterior insertion of the deltoid ligament.
8. The tendons of the neurovascular bundle are retracted, exposing a mass of scar tissue composed of the posterior tibial tendon, the superficial deltoid ligament, the capsule of the talonavicular joint, and the spring ligament. The navicular will be found displaced medially to the head of the talus.
9. Mobilization of the navicular is initiated by dividing the posterior tibial tendon and excising the mass of scar tissue.
10. Accomplish the medial release by returning to the side of the posterior release and everting the foot, thus exposing the subtalar joint.
11. Now release the superficial layer of the deltoid ligament from the calcaneus. (The deep portion must not be excised, to prevent flatfoot.)
12. Next the subtalar release completes the mobilization of the anterior end of the calcaneus and the navicular. The talocalcaneal interosseous ligament is exposed by everting the foot and is transected. Mobilization of the navicular is completed by transecting the bifurcate ligament, which extends from the calcaneus to the lateral border of the navicular and to the medial border of the cuboid.
13. Divide the distal remnant of the posterior tibial tendon.
14. After the contractures are released, reduce the deformity without force. When the navicular is reduced onto the head of the talus, the other tarsal bones are carried with it.
15. Insert a Kirschner wire in the region of the first metatarsal, transfixing the talonavicular joint. Resuture the Achilles tendon to allow dorsiflexion to a right angle. Avoid excessive lengthening which increases atrophy of the calf muscles.
16. Close all wounds in layers and apply an above-knee cast with the knee in slight flexion.
17. Post-op care includes immobilization for four months, followed by protection in a Dennis Browne splint with a 25 cm crossbar that the child wears during his sleeping hours for one year. Lateral sole wedges are used during the day for two years after cast removal.

---

incised, and medial and dorsal aspects of talonavicular joint have been opened. (G) View of posteromedial aspect of subtalar joint. Tibiocalcaneal part of deltoid ligament has been divided, but tibiotalar part has not. Flexor hallucis longus tendon is to be freed from its sheath and retracted posteriorly and medial talocalcaneal ligament is to be divided, allowing calcaneus to be fully everted. (Reproduced with permision from Gelman, W.B. In A.F. DePalma (Ed.): *Clinical Orthopaedics*, Vol. 16, J.B. Lippincott, Philadelphia, 1960, p. 179.)

Gelman Technique[6]

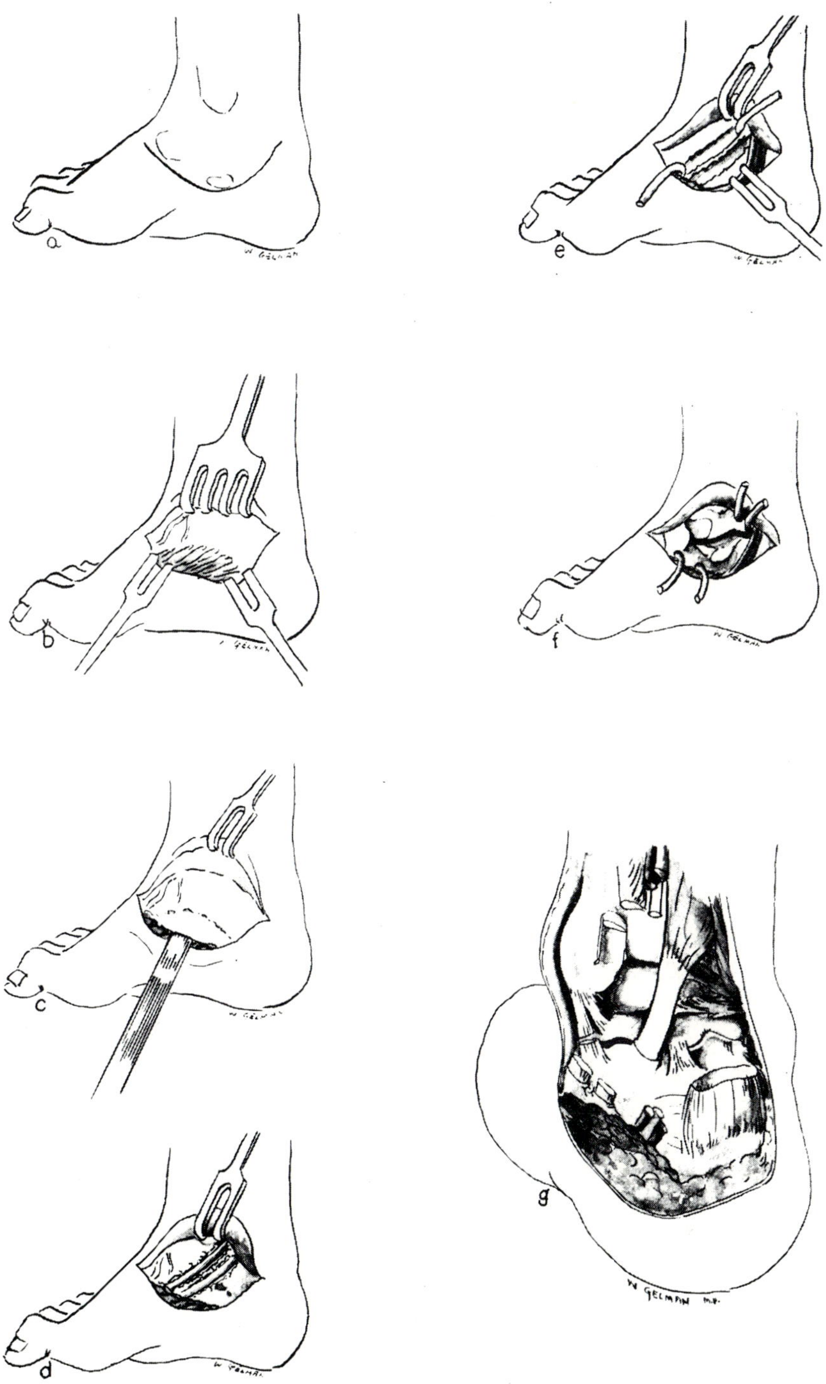

Figure 2. Gelman soft tissue releasing operation. (A) Incision. (B) Abductor hallucis muscle has been exposed. (C) Abductor hallucis has been freed and retracted plantarward. (D) Sheaths of tibialis posterior and flexor digitorum longus tendons have been incised. (E) Tibialis posterior tendon has been divided by Z-plasty, and flexor digitorum longus tendon and neurovascular bundle have been retracted posteriorly. (F) Tibiocalcaneal part of deltoid ligament has been divided, medial part of capsule of subtalar joint has been

(legend continued on facing page)

1. Make a curved incision convex plantarward beginning at the Achilles tendon, passing anteriorly just inferior to the sustentaculum tali, and ending at the first cuneiform.
2. Deepen and expose the abductor hallucis muscle and free it.
3. Incise the sheaths of the tibialis posterior and flexor digitorum longus tendons. Divide the tibialis posterior by Z-plasty and retract the flexor digitorum posteriorly.
4. Divide the tibiocalcaneal part of the deltoid ligament preserving the tibiotalar part; at this point the subtalar joint should be open at the sustentaculum tali.
5. Incise the medial aspect of the subtalar capsule and the thickened capsule of the talonavicular joint that binds the sustentaculum tali and the tuberosity of the navicular to the medial malleolus.
6. Next free the posterior part of the subtalar joint medially by transecting the flexor hallucis longus tendon, the medial talocalcaneal ligaments, and the interosseous talocalcaneal ligaments.
7. Post-op care as previously described.

Bost Technique[6]

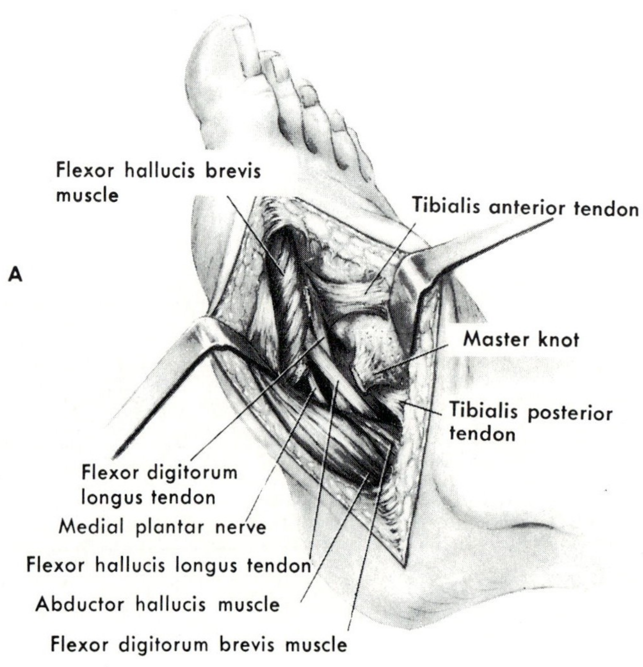

Figure 3. (Reproduced with permission from Crenshaw, A.H. (Ed.): *Campbell's Operative Orthopaedics*, Vol. 2, C.V. Mosby, St. Louis, 1971, p. 1914.) *Continued on facing page.*

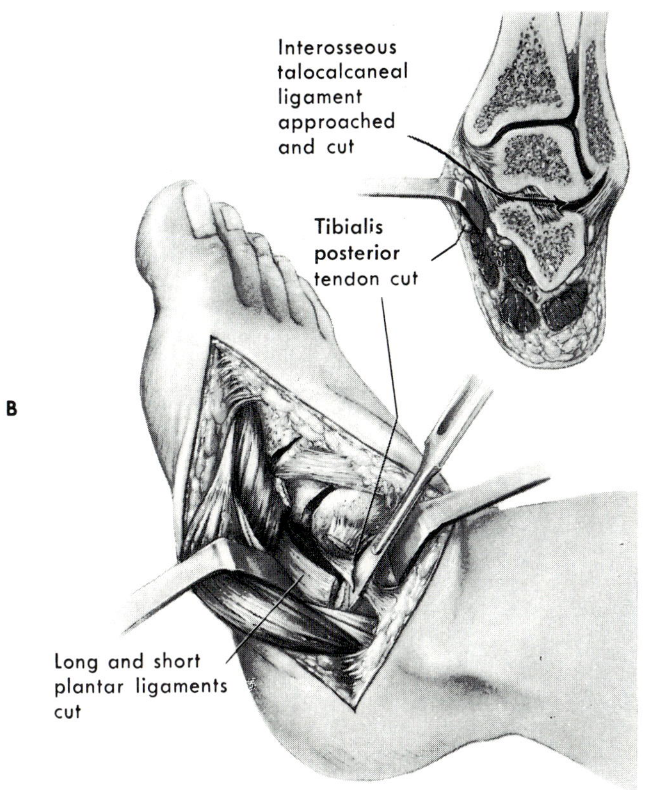

Figure 3 (continued). (Reproduced with permission from Crenshaw, A.H. (Ed.): *Campbell's Operative Orthopaedics*, Vol. 2, C.V. Mosby, St. Louis, 1971, p. 1914.)

1. Make a medial incision convex dorsally, beginning posteriorly at the medial aspect of the tuberosity of the calcaneus continuing distally along the navicular and ending at the proximal phalanx of the great toe.
2. Free the abductor hallucis posteriorly to the medial aspect of the calcaneal tuberosity and retract it plantarly.
3. Divide the "Master Knot" of Henry and free the flexor digitorum longus and flexor hallucis longus tendons from the plantar of the navicular.
4. Divide the origin of the flexor hallucis brevis and retract all plantar intrinsic muscles.
5. Now free the posterior tibial tendon from the navicular, first cuneiform and metatarsals. Also free the plantar intrinsic muscles from the tuberosity of the calcaneus.
6. At the calcaneocuboid joint, divide the long and short plantar ligaments and the plantar aspect of the capsule of this joint.
7. Divide the ligaments of the talocalcaneonavicular joint. Transect the deltoid ligament from the navicular, the medial margin of the calcaneonavicular ligament, the sustentaculum tali, and the medial side of the talus.
8. Next divide the medial talocalcaneal ligaments, the anterior capsule of the subtalar joint and the interosseous talocalcaneal ligaments. Incise the

medial navicular-cuneiform joint on its medial and plantar aspects and extend the plantar incision to free the navicular from the second and third cuneiforms.

9. Retract the tibialis anterior tendon and divide the first metatarsal-cuneiform joint capsules.
10. Put the foot in corrected position, reattach the abductor hallucis muscle to the fascia, and apply a long leg cast.
11. Post-op care as previously discussed.

Garceau Technique[6]

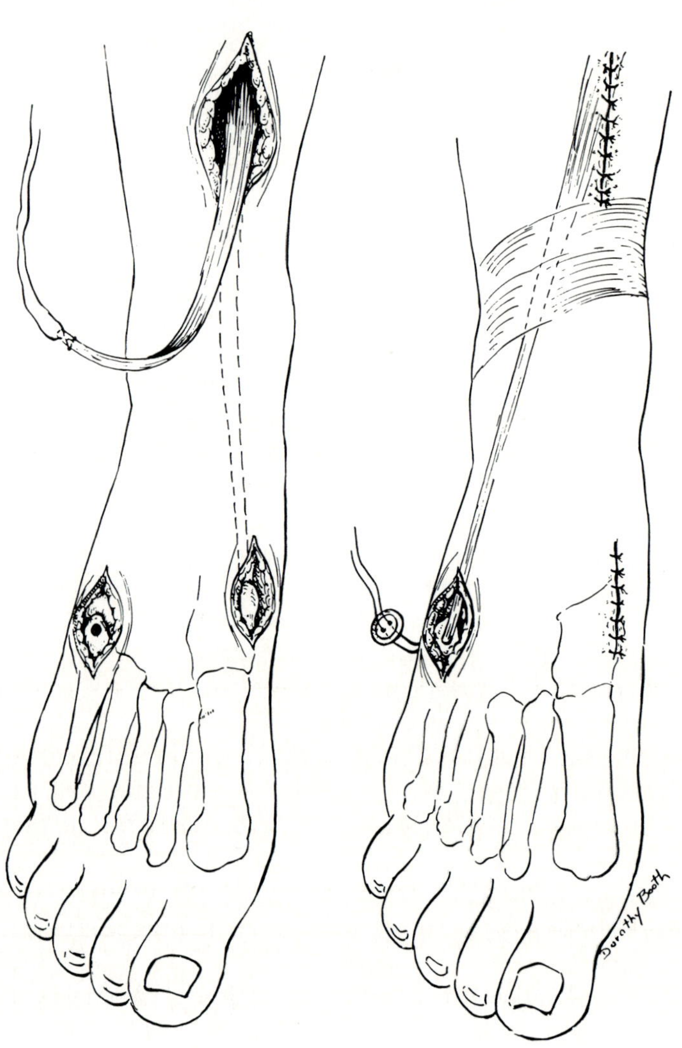

Figure 4. (Reproduced with permission from Carpenter, E.B., and Huff, S.H.: *Southern Medical Journal*, **46**:220, 1953.)

1. Make a 1 inch incision over the tibialis anterior tendon just proximal to the ankle.
2. Make a second longitudinal incision over the first cuneiform, and expose and free the insertion of the tendon, pulling it out of the proximal incision.
3. Next pass a hemostat from the proximal incision distally beneath the cruciate crural ligament to the base of the fifth metatarsal. At this point expose the fifth metatarsal through a third incision and drill a hole in it.
4. Now place a suture through the tibialis anterior tendon and pass it through the drill hole and anchor it.
5. Immobilize in a short leg cast for eight weeks, after which muscle re-education should be continued.

References

1. Goldstein, L.A., and Dickerson, R.C.: *Atlas of Orthopaedic Surgery*, C.V. Mosby, St. Louis, 1974, p. 913.
2. Gelman, W.B.: Soft tissue releasing procedure for persisting heel varus in the uncorrected clubfoot. *Clin. Orthoped.*, **16**:177, 1960.
3. Bost, F.C.: Plantar dissection. An operation to release the soft tissues in recurrent or recalcitrant talipes equino varus. *J. Bone Jt. Surg.*, **42-A**:151, 1960.
4. Turco, V.J.: Surgical correction of the resistant club foot. One stage posteromedial release with internal fixation. *J. Bone Jt. Surg.*, **53-A**:477, 1971.
5. Garceau, G.J.: Anterior tibial transposition in recurrent congenital club foot. *J. Bone Jt. Surg.*, **22**:932, 1940.
6. Crenshaw, A.H. (Ed.): *Campbell's Operative Orthopaedics*, Vol. 2, C.V. Mosby, St. Louis, 1971.

Selected Bibliography

Brockman, E.P.: Modern methods of treatment of clubfoot. *Br. Med. J.*, **2**:512, 1937.

Carpenter, E.B.: Selective tendon transfers for recurrent clubfoot. *South. Med. J.*, **46**:220, 1953.

Evans, D.: Relapsed club foot. *J. Bone Jt. Surg.*, **43-B**:722, 1961.

Fripp, A.T.: Recurrent congenital club foot. The tole of the M. Tibilias posterior in etiology and treatment. *J. Bone Jt. Surg.*, **41-A**:243, 1959.

Gartland, J.J.: Posterior tibial transplant in the surgical treatment of recurrent club foot. A preliminary report. *J. Bone Jt. Surg.*, **46A**:1217, 1964.

Kite, J.H.: The surgical treatment of congenital club foot. Surg. *Gynecol. Obstet.*, **61**:190, 1935.

McCauley, J.C., Jr.: A release operation for problem club foot. *N.Y. J. Med.* **52**:2997, 1952.

Tachdjian, M.O.: *Pediatric Orthopedics*, Vol. II, W.B. Saunders Company, Philadelphia, 1972, pp. 1295-1315.

Turco, V.J.: Surgical correction of the resistant congenital club foot — one-stage release with internal fixation. *A.A.O.S. Film Library*.

Turco, V.J.: Surgical correction of the resistant clubfoot. One-stage posteromedial release with internal fixation: A preliminary report. *J. Bone Jt. Surg.*, **53-A**:477, 1971.

Wagner, L.C., and Butterfield, W.L.: Surgical release of contracted tissues for resistant congenital club foot. *Am. J. Surg.*, **84**:82, 1952.

CHAPTER 19

Tarsal Tunnel Syndrome

Tarsal tunnel syndrome is among the peripheral entrapment neuropathies associated with mechanical factors that involve the peripheral nerve in bony and fibromuscular tissues. In the tarsal tunnel syndrome, compression on the tibial nerve causes diffuse, intermittent sharp pain in the

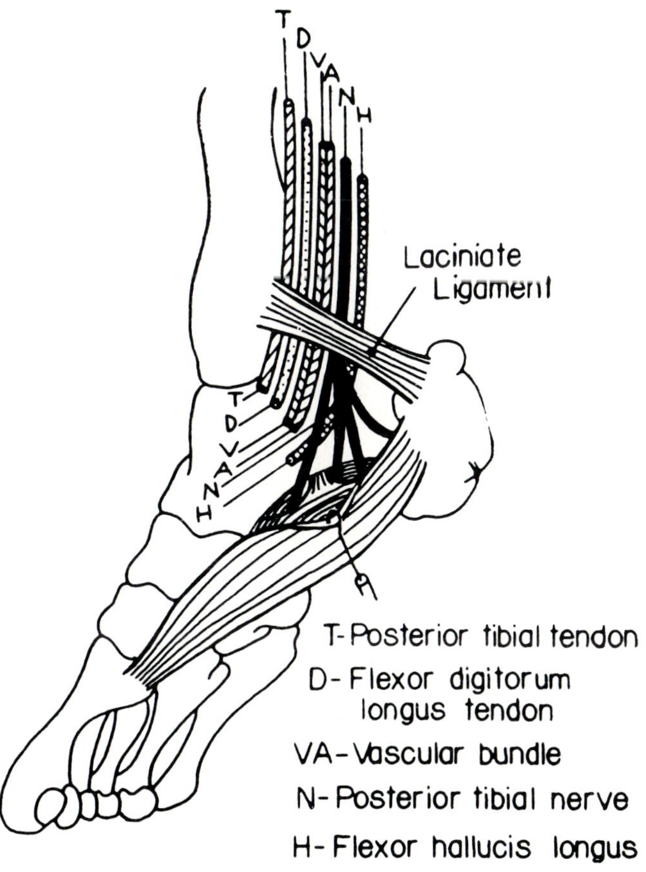

Figure 1. The "Tarsal Tunnel". Note arrangement of structures beneath the laciniate ligament. The posterior tibial nerve can be easily trapped particularly following an ankle fracture with excess callus formation or any other space-occupying cause in this area. (Reproduced with permission from Giannestras, N.J.: *Foot Disorders: Medical and Surgical Management,* Lea & Febiger, Philadelphia, 1967, p. 366.)

plantar aspect of the foot where the nerve passes behind and beneath the tibial malleolus.[1] Compression of the nerve also produces paresthesis of the toes, and the symptoms may be more acute at night. The patient will complain of numbness and tingling in the sole of the foot and the toes, followed by burning pain in the ankle. In chronic cases, motor and sensory impairment may result in paresis or paralysis of the small muscles of the foot.

Diagnosis

The diagnosis of tarsal tunnel syndrome relies on six factors or tests:

1. A positive Hoffman-Tinel sign will be elicited by direct pressure over the flexor reticulum and tarsal tunnel region. This sign is characterized by tingling in the area of the distribution of the nerve and numbness in the toes. It is a quantitative index of sensory fiber regeneration.
2. Direct pressure will produce nerve trunk tenderness above and below the point of compression (valleix phenomenon).
3. Application of a venous tourniquet to the lower limb will elicit symptoms of venous occlusion—transient passive congestion and ischemia.
4. Forced inversion or eversion of the foot will produce increased numbness, particularly when the hallux joint is flexed.
5. Electromyographic study will reveal increased distal latencies from a stimulation point above the medial malleolus to either the abductor hallucis or the abductor digiti quinti.
6. Injection of 2 ml of 1% lidocaine to block the distal tibial nerve will elicit relief for up to two hours. It must be cautioned, however, that this is not necessarily indicative of tarsal tunnel syndrome, and a differential diagnosis is necessary to rule out distal lesions in the foot as a cause of the symptoms being considered.

Treatment

Conservative treatment of tarsal tunnel syndrome involves corticosteroid injection with local anesthetic to block the posterior tibial nerve. The patient then wears a flexible cast (unna boot). In some cases it may be advisable to use an orthotic appliance to limit pronation.

If conservative means fail, operation to free the tibial nerve from surrounding tissue will be necessary. The procedure involves decompression by release of the flexor reticulum and all fibrous bands that are constricting the nerve.

Kuritz and Sokoloff Technique[2]

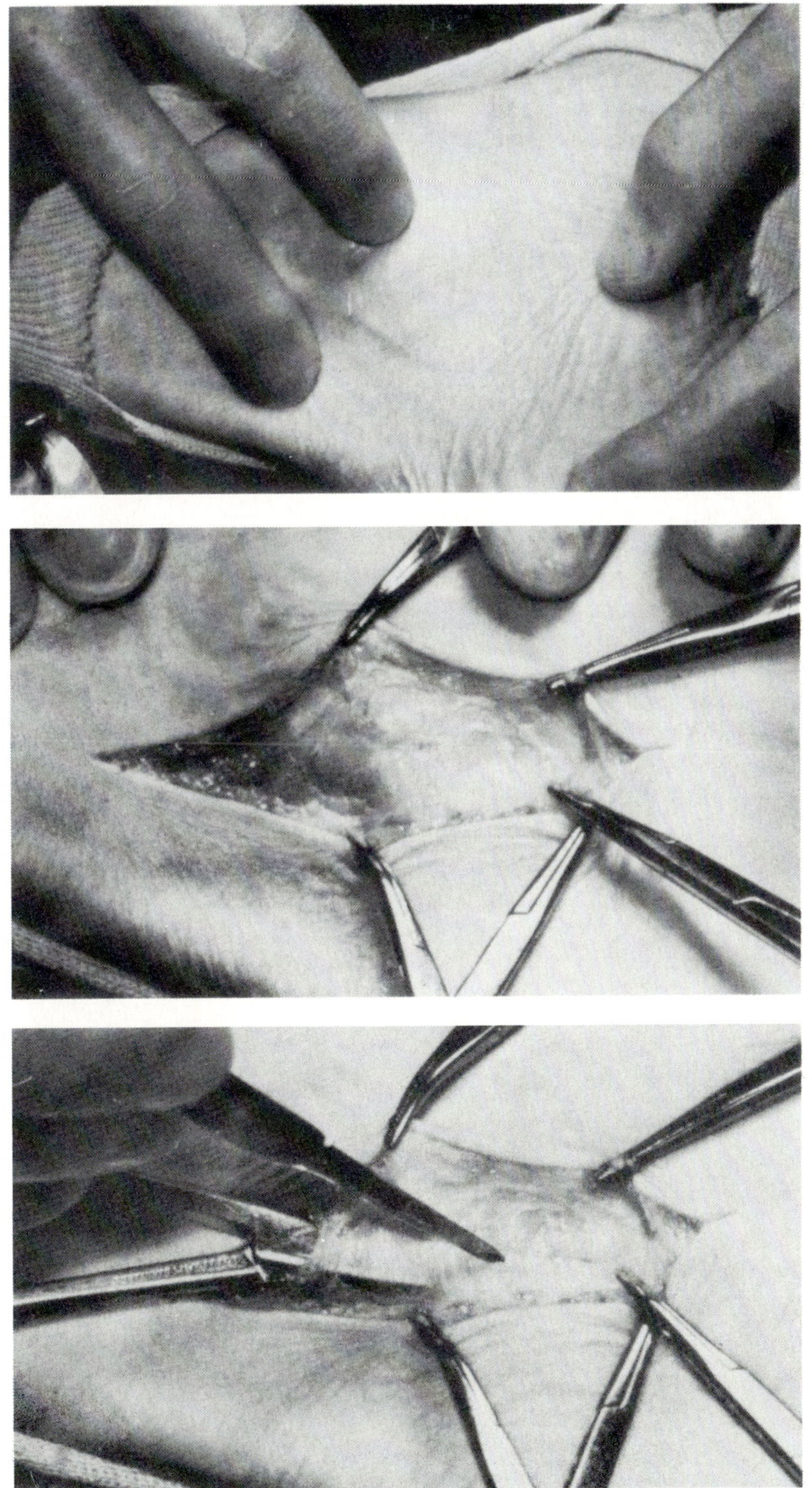

Figure 2. (Reproduced with permission from Kuritz, A., and Sokoloff, T.: Tarsal tunnel syndrome, *J. Am. Pod. Assoc.*, **65**:833–839, 1975.) *Continued on following page.*

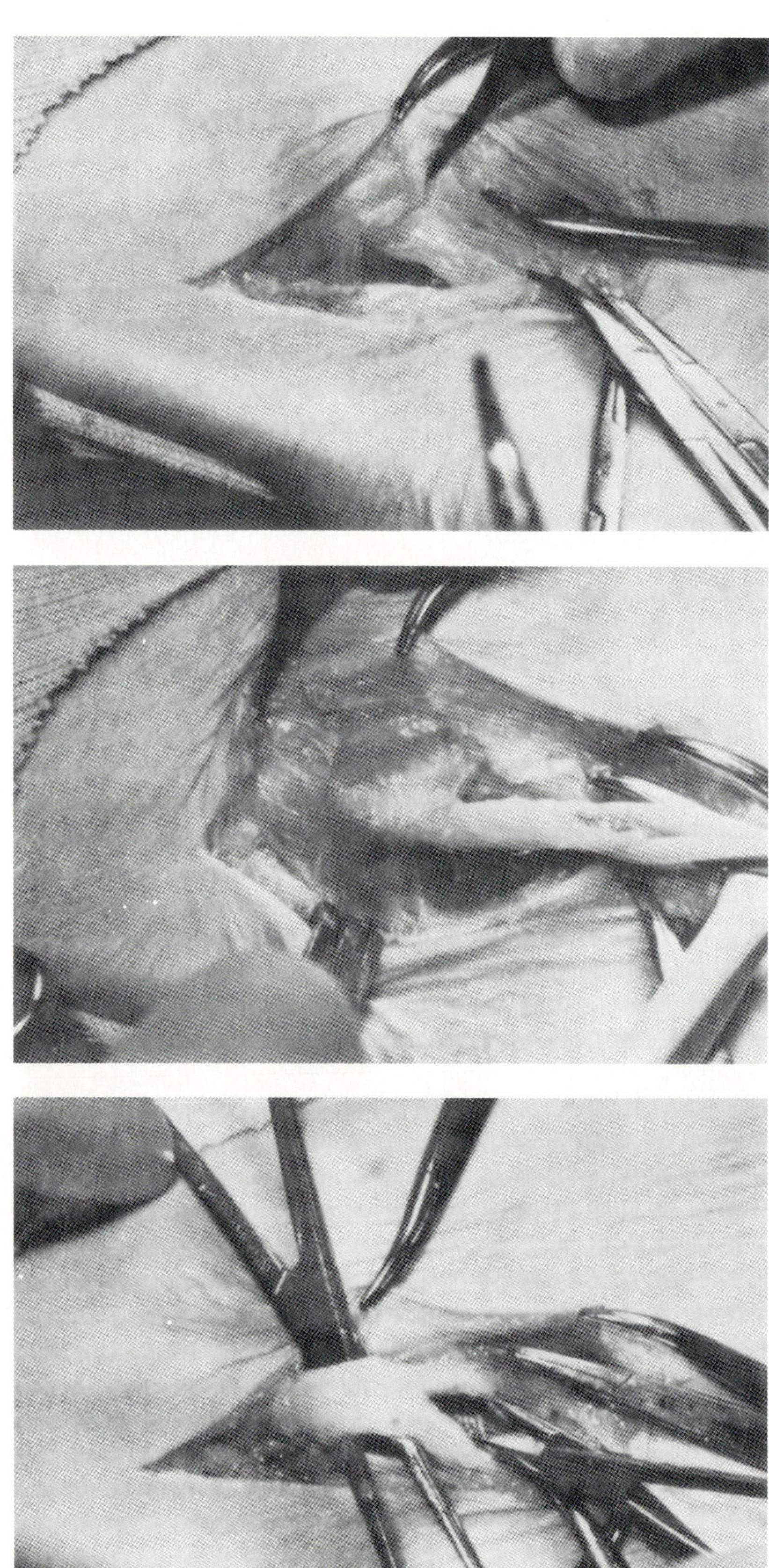

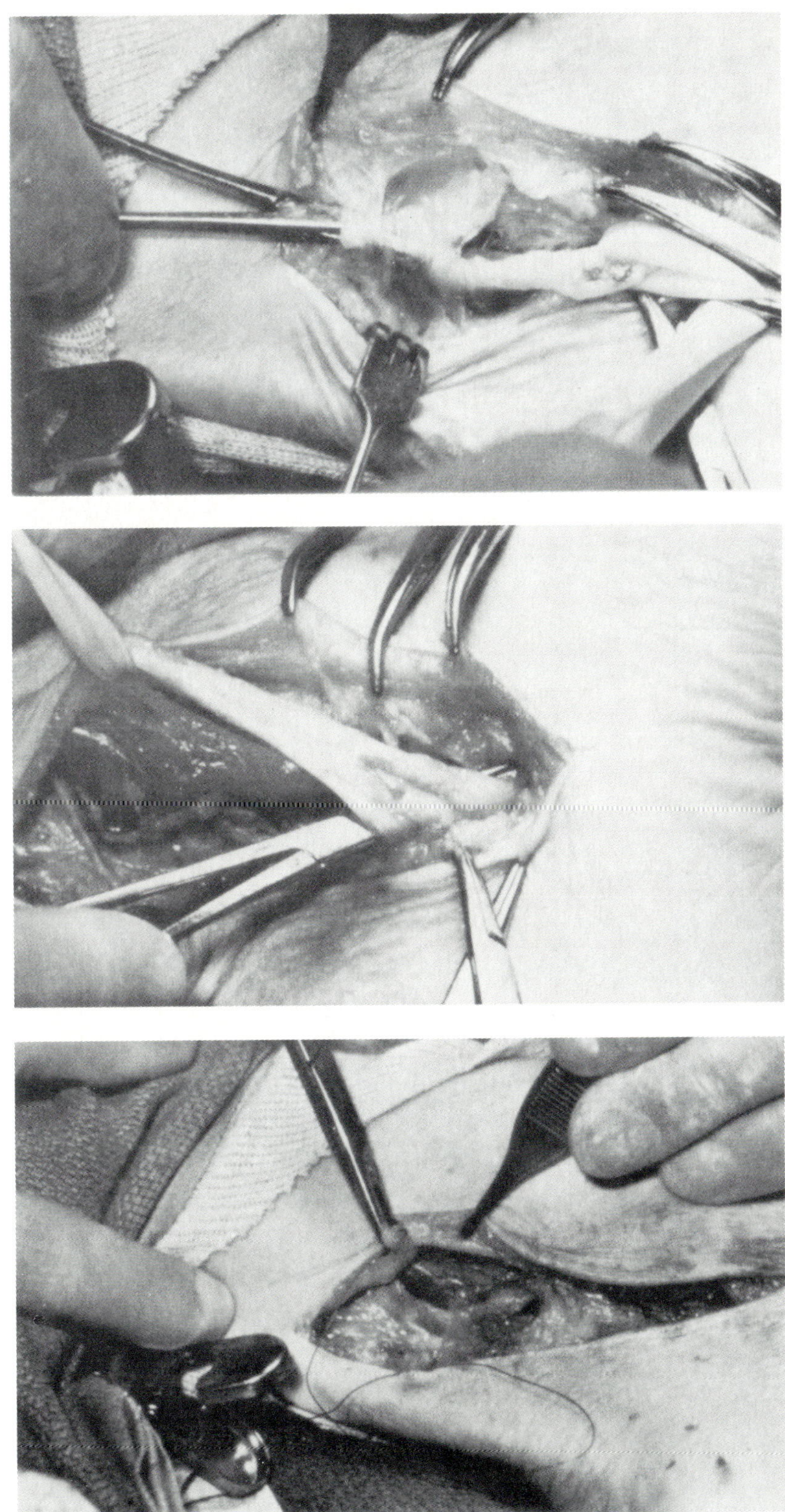

Figure 2 (continued). (Reproduced with permission from Kuritz, A., and Sokoloff, T.: Tarsal tunnel syndrome, *J. Am. Pod. Assoc.*, **65**:833–839, 1975.) *Continued on following page.*

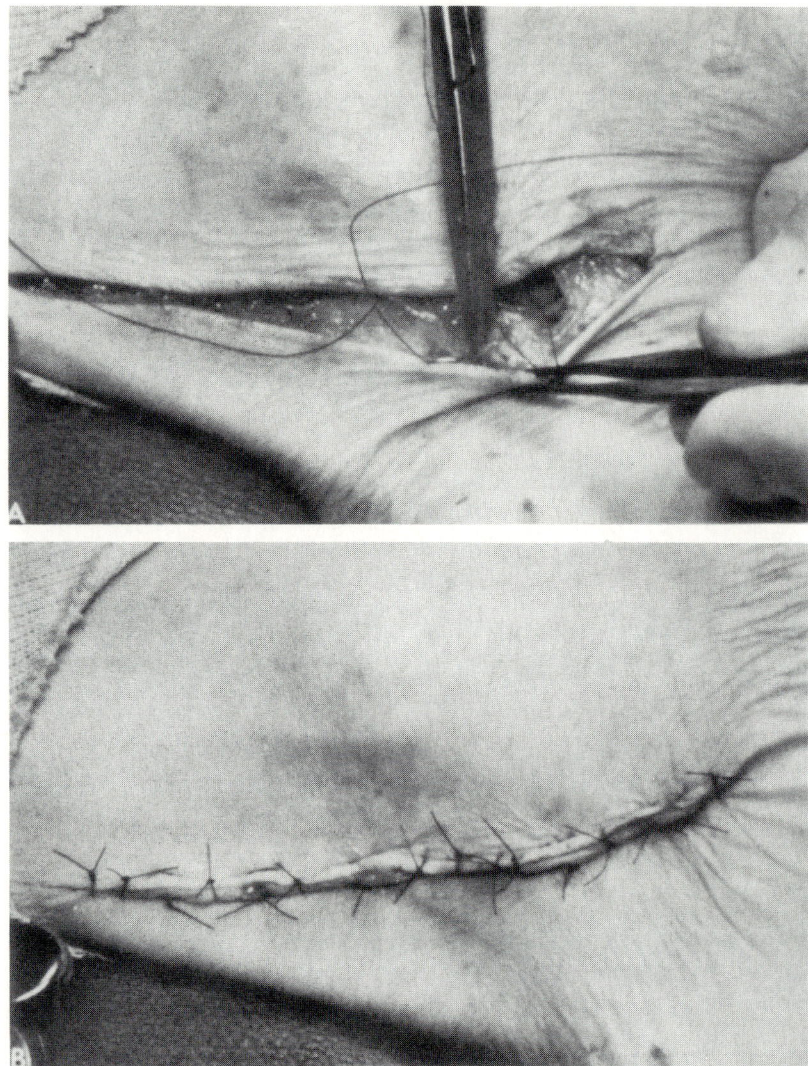

Figure 2 (continued). (Reproduced with permission from Kuritz, A., and Sokoloff, T.: Tarsal tunnel syndrome, *J. Am. Pod. Assoc.*, **65**:833–839, 1975.)

1. A curvilinear incision is made posteromedially, beginning at a point several centimeters proximal to the medial malleolus and continuing distally along the course of the posterior tibial nerve, behind and below the medial malleolus (A).
2. Through sharp and blunt dissection, the subcutaneous tissue is incised and the neurovascular structures superior to the retinaculum are identified and retracted laterally (B).
3. Care should be taken to visualize the calcaneal branch, which may pierce the flexor retinaculum at this level (C).
4. The flexor retinaculum is incised and the posterior tibial nerve is identified, mobilized, and retracted with a penrose drain to avoid trauma (D,E).
5. The nerve is followed proximally, incising the flexor retinaculum, and

distally to a point where the medial and lateral branches pass through the fibrous canals superior to the abductor hallucis muscle belly (F).

6. Examination of the posterior tibial vein may reveal varicosity and this should be ligated and excised. The abductor hallucis is examined for hypertrophy, and hypertrophic tissue may be excised (G,H).
7. The superficial fascia, only, is approximated with absorbable suture of choice (I).
8. The flexor retinaculum is not approximated with deep suture closure (J).
9. Incision closed in the usual manner (K).
10. Sterile dressing and a below-the-knee walking cast are applied for immobilization. Cast and sutures are removed after three weeks, and the patient is allowed to increase activities gradually. Approximately six months after decompression, nerve conduction studies may be done to follow the nerve healing process.

References

1. Giannestras, N.J.: *Foot Disorders: Medical and Surgical Management*, Lea & Febiger, Philadelphia, 1967.
2. Kuritz, A., and Sokoloff, T.: Tarsal tunnel syndrome. *J. Am. Pod. Assoc.*, **65**:825–839, 1975.
3. Levin, H.: The tarsal tunnel syndrome. *J. Foot Surg.*, **13**:59–62, 1974.

Selected Bibliography

Chater, E.H., and Wilson, A.L.: Tarsal tunnel syndrome. *J. Irish Med. Assoc.*, **61**:326–328, 1968.

Crenshaw, A.H. (Ed.): *Campbell's Operative Orthopaedics*, Vol. 2, C.V. Mosby, St. Louis, 1963.

Dickerson, L.A., and Goldstein, R.C.: *Atlas of Orthopaedic Surgery*, Vol. 2, C.V. Mosby, St. Louis, 1974.

Distefano, V.: Tarsal tunnel syndrome. *Clin. Orthoped.*, **88**:76–79, 1972.

Edwards, W.G., Lincoln, C.R., Basset, F.H., III et al.: The tarsal tunnel syndrome. Diagnosis and treatment. *J.A.M.A.*, **207**:716, 1969.

Inman, V.T. (Ed.): *DuVries' Surgery of the Foot*, 3 ed., C.V. Mosby, St. Louis, 1973.

McGlamry, E.D.: *Reconstructive Surgery of the Foot and Leg*, Intercontinental Medical Book Corp., New York, 1974.

McGlone, J.J.: The tarsal tunnel syndrome. *J. Am. Pod. Assoc.*, **58**:435–437, 1968.

Ward, W.C.: Posterior tibial nerve injuries. *Surgery*, **14**:124–129, 1948.

CHAPTER 20

Tarsal Coalition

Coalition between two or more tarsal bones may be congenital or acquired. Regardless of the etiology, the union may be characteristically osseous (synostosis), cartilaginous (synchondrosis), or fibrous (syndesmosis). The nature and degree of the coalition may also vary from moderate to extreme. The most common forms are the talocalcaneal bridge and the calcaneonavicular, talonavicular, and calcaneocuboid bar.

In children, symptoms generally do not begin until the second decade of life, when the ossification of fibrous or cartilaginous bars begins. As bony tissue develops, subtalar and midtarsal articulation becomes progressively restricted; in adults, tarsal coalition can lead to the very painful rigid flatfoot.

The several forms of tarsal coalition produce varying degrees of foot valgus, and mild forms are sometimes overlooked. For the most part, a calcaneonavicular union will produce less deformation than a talocalcaneal bridge.

Roentgenographic studies of calcaneonavicular coalition will reveal irregularities of the cortical bone surfaces at their junction. The talar head may be hypoplastic and underdeveloped. If the bar or bridge is fibrous or cartilaginous, the bone irregularities will be indistinct, so it is advisable to take x-ray studies at a 45 degree oblique angle. Likewise, a talocalcaneal coalition may be difficult to identify roentgenographically because the subtalar joint is a complex structure. Lateral oblique and axial projections afford the best views of lateral beaking at the head of the talus, broadening of the lateral talar process, and narrowing of the posterior talocalcaneal facet. Talonavicular coalition is readily evident on an anteroposterior x-ray film, which will reveal absence of the joint.

The course of therapy depends upon the clinical symptoms and severity of deformity. The adolescent with tarsal coalition symptomatology, and no radiographic proof, should be treated for six weeks with sinus tarsi steroid injections and a short leg walking cast. If the symptomatology is excessive, the cast should be applied in a pronatory direction thereby relieving the already spastic peroneal group. The surgeon must make every conservative effort to relieve symptoms until the individual reaches osseous maturity; however, a Grice-Green extra-articular arthrodesis may be necessary to relieve pain.

Calcaneonavicular bar may be resected successfully before complete ossification of the bar. Cowell recommends bar excision and extensor brevis arthroplasty in a patient under fourteen years of age who has pain in the foot, limited subtalar joint motion, and a cartilaginous bar. It should not be performed in the presence of degenerative changes in the talonavicular joint with accompanying talar beak, or when there is a concomitant talocalcaneal bar. Tachdjian is also in complete agreement; however, he will perform the procedure beyond fourteen years of age.

If adaptive or degenerative changes have already occurred at the subtalar and midtarsal joints, tarsal resection is contraindicated and may lead to total joint instability. The treatment of choice in this case is triple arthrodesis.

In talocalcaneal coalition, treatment is directed at the stabilization of the foot. Bar resection will only create an unstable valgus positioned foot without restoring subtalar joint motion. As a result, talocalcaneal coalition lends itself to a triple arthrodesis procedure. If there is complete ossification of the medial talocalcaneal bar, then an arthrodesis of the talonavicular joint may be helpful in preventing gross deformity and pain. Talonavicular and calcaneocuboid bars require no treatment as symptomatology is rare and easily corrected by conservative measures.

Excision of Calcaneonavicular Bar

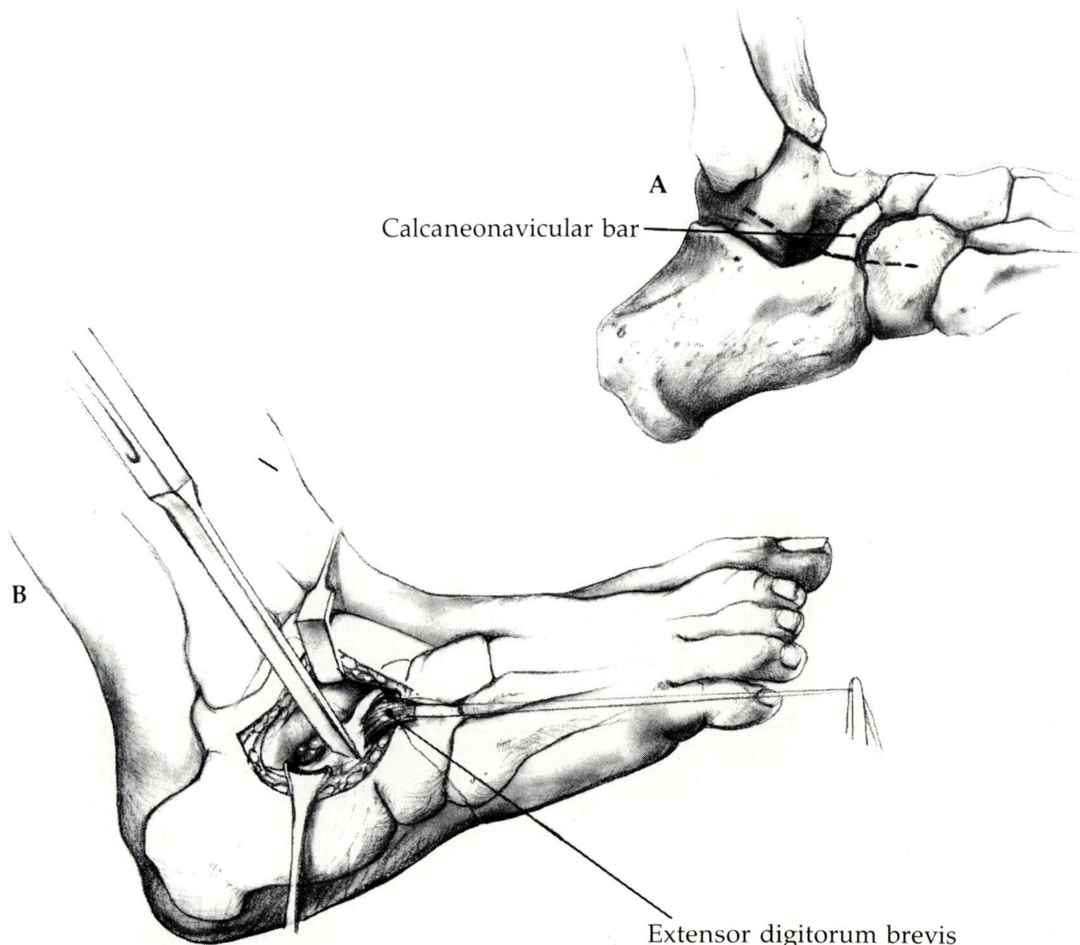

Figure 1. (Reproduced with permission from Goldstein, L.A., and Dickerson, R.C.:*Atlas of Orthopaedic Surgery*, Vol. 2, C.V. Mosby, St. Louis, 1974, p. 931.) *Continued on facing page.*

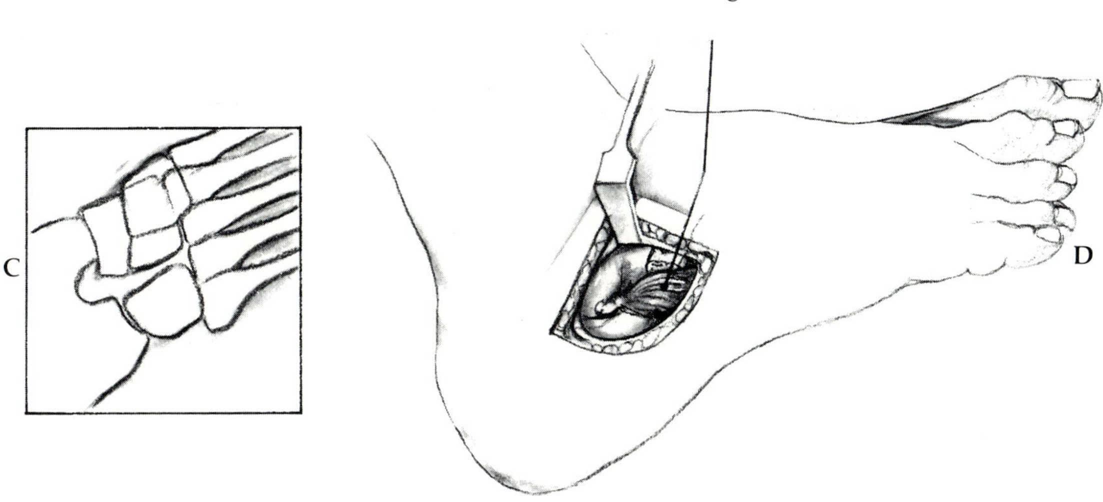

Figure 1 (continued). (Reproduced with permission from Goldstein, L.A., and Dickerson, R.C.: *Atlas of Orthopaedic Surgery*, Vol. 2, C.V. Mosby, St. Louis, 1974, p. 931.)

1. A lateral Ollier incision is used, extending from a point just below the fibula malleolus forward toward the calcaneocuboid joint.
2. Carry the dissection down to expose the origin of the extensor digitorum brevis muscle, which is reflected distally.
3. The calcaneocuboid and talonavicular joints are opened sufficiently to expose the calcaneonavicular bar.
4. An osteotome is then used to divide the calcaneal and navicular ends of the bar. The entire bar is removed as a rectangle, not a wedge. The osteotome is almost horizontal in dividing the calcaneal portion of the bar. The osteotome is angled downward as the navicular portion of the bar is divided.
5. The bony synostosis is removed and the raw cancellous bleeding bases of the excised bar are coagulated.
6. The origin of the extensor brevis digitorum is then sutured into the defect formerly occupied by the synostosis. Two Keith needles are used on each side of the suture; the needles are pulled out on the medial side of the foot, where the suture is tied over a well-padded bottom.
7. The wound is closed and the foot immobilized in a short leg cast. The cast is bivalved in approximately ten days, so that passive and active inversion and eversion of the hindfoot may be begun.
8. Full weight-bearing usually requires eight weeks.

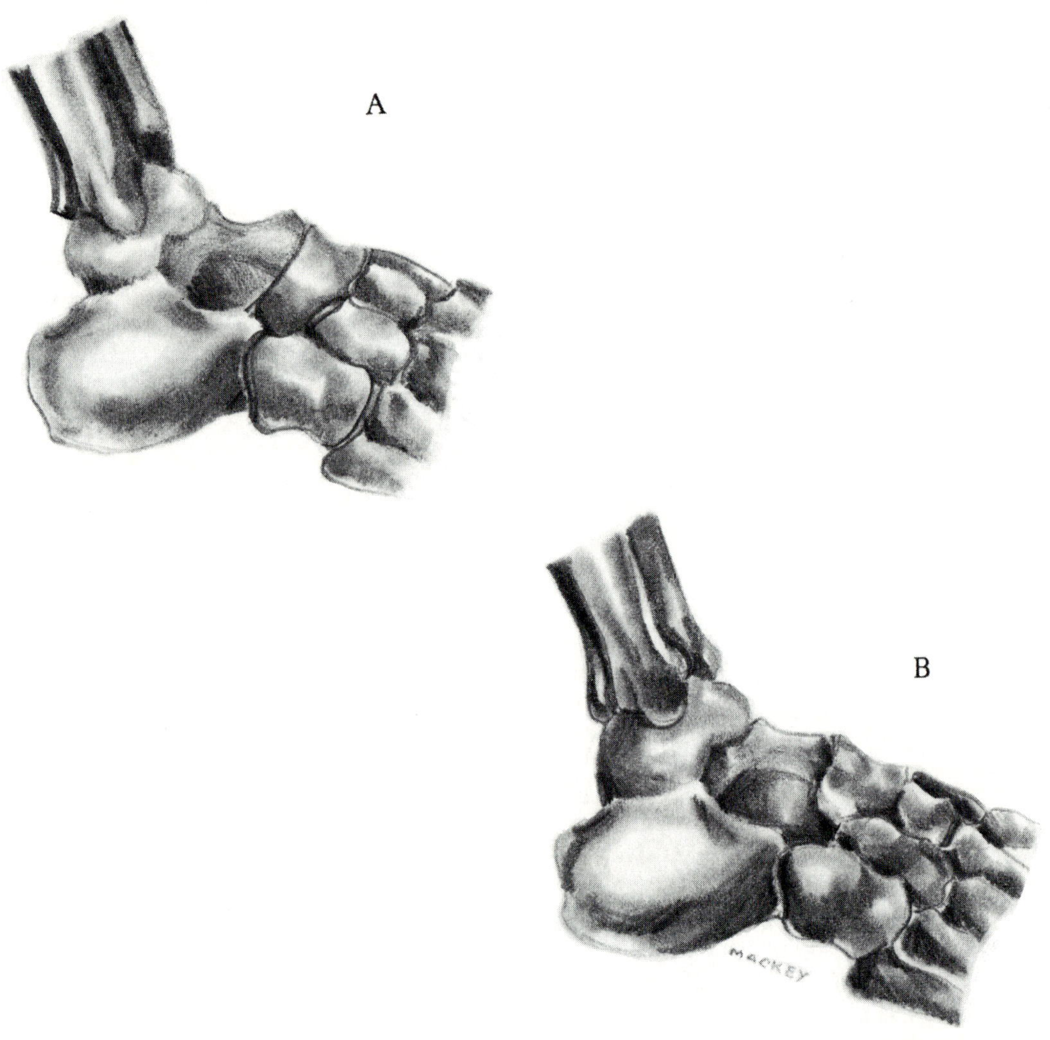

Figure 2. Calcaneonavicular bar. (A) Before excision of bar. (B) After excision of bar.

References

1. Goldstein, L.A., and Dickerson, R.C.: *Atlas of Orthopaedic Surgery*, C.V. Mosby, St. Louis, 1974.

Selected Bibliography

Bagley, O.D.: A critical analysis of tarsal coalitions. *Arch. Pod. Med. & Foot Surg.*, **I**,3:195–208, 1974.

Bersani, F.A., and Samilton, R.L.: Massive familial tarsal synostosis. *J. Bone Jt. Surg.*, **39-A**:1187, 1957.

Blockley, N.J.: Peroneal spastic flat foot. *J. Bone Jt. Surg.*, **37-B**:191, 1955.

Conway, J.J., and Cowell, H.R.: Tarsal coalition: Clinical significance and roentgenographic demonstration. *Radiology*, **92**:799, 1969.

Cowell, H.R.: Extensor brevis arthroplasty. *J. Bone Jt. Surg.*, **52-A**:820, 1970.

DePalma, A.F.: *Clinical Orthopedics*, J.B. Lippincott, Phildelphia, 1960.

Gaynor, S.S.: Congenital astragalocalcaneal fusion. *J. Bone Jt. Surg.*, **18**:479, 1936.

Hark, F.W.: Congenital anomalies of the tarsal bones. *Clin. Orthoped.*, **16**:21–25, 1960.

Harris, R.I., and Beath, T.: Ethology of peroneal spastic flat foot. *J. Bone Jt. Surg.*, **30-B**:624, 1948.

Jack, E.A.: Bone anomalies of the tarsus in relation to peroneal spastic flat foot. *J. Bone Jt. Surg.*, **36-B**:530–542, 1954.

Kaplan, E.G., and Kaplan, G.S.: Tarsal coalition: Review and preliminary conclusions. *J. Foot Surg.*, **15**:136–143, 1977.

Lapidus, P.W.: Spastic flat foot. *J. Bone Jt. Surg.*, **28**:126, 1946.

Outland, T., and Murphy, I.O.: The pathomechanics of peroneal spastic flat foot. *Clin. Orthoped.*, **16**:64–73, 1960.

Sanghi, J.K., and Roby, H.R.: Bilateral peroneal spastic flat foot associated with congenital fusion to the navicular and talus. *J. Bone Jt. Surg.*, **43A**:1237, 1961.

Stoller, M.I.: Tarsal coalition: Study of surgical results. *J.A.P.A.*, 1004, 1974.

Tachdjian, M.O.: *Pediatric Orthopaedics*, Vol. 2, W.B. Saunders, Philadelphia, 1972.

Webster, F.S., and Roberts, E.M.: Tarsal anomalies and peroneal spastic flat foot, *J.A.M.A.*, **146**:1099–1104, 1951.

Index